Tibia Pathology and Fractures

Edited by Dimitrios D. Nikolopoulos, George K. Safos and John Michos

Published in London, United Kingdom

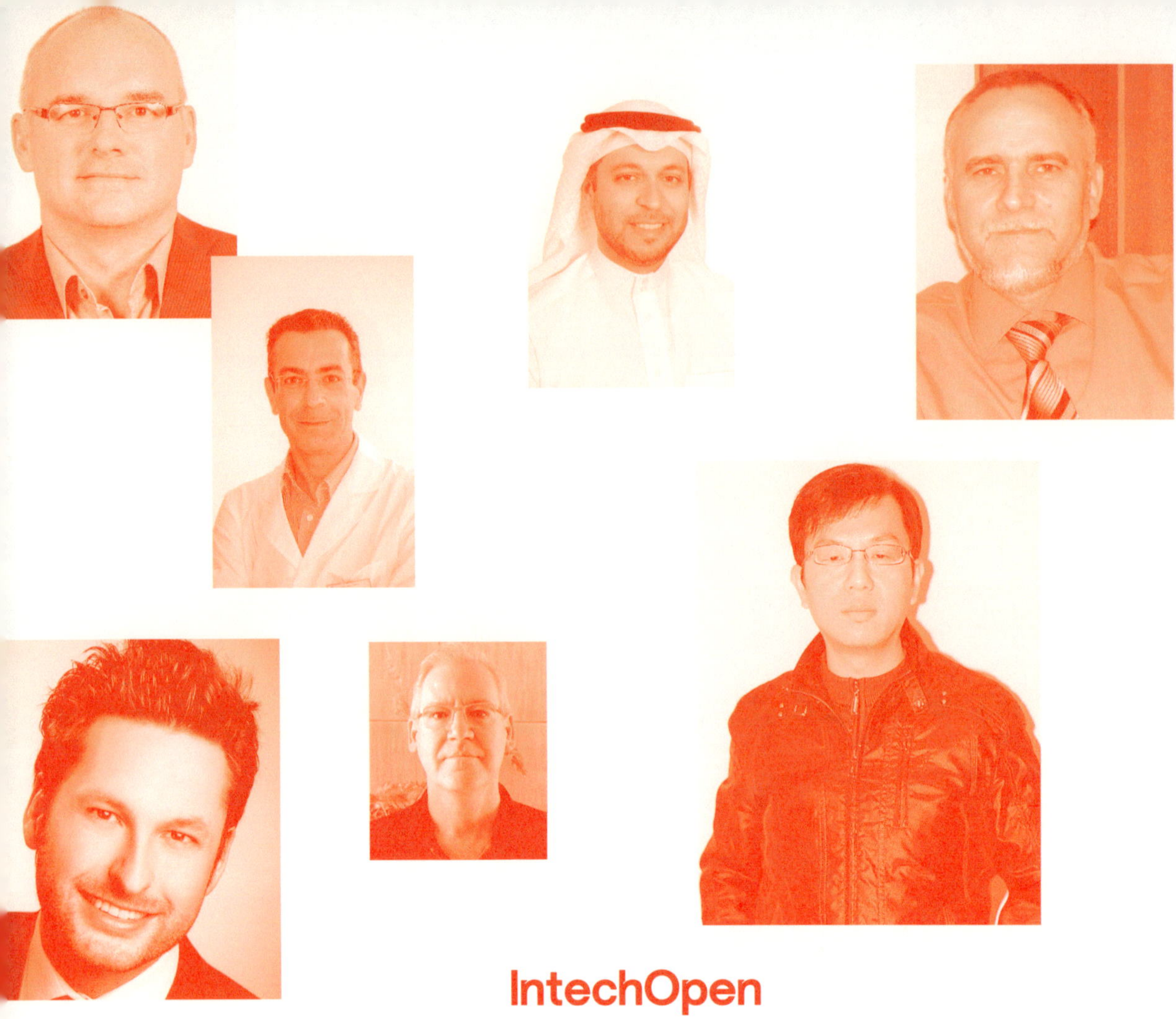

IntechOpen

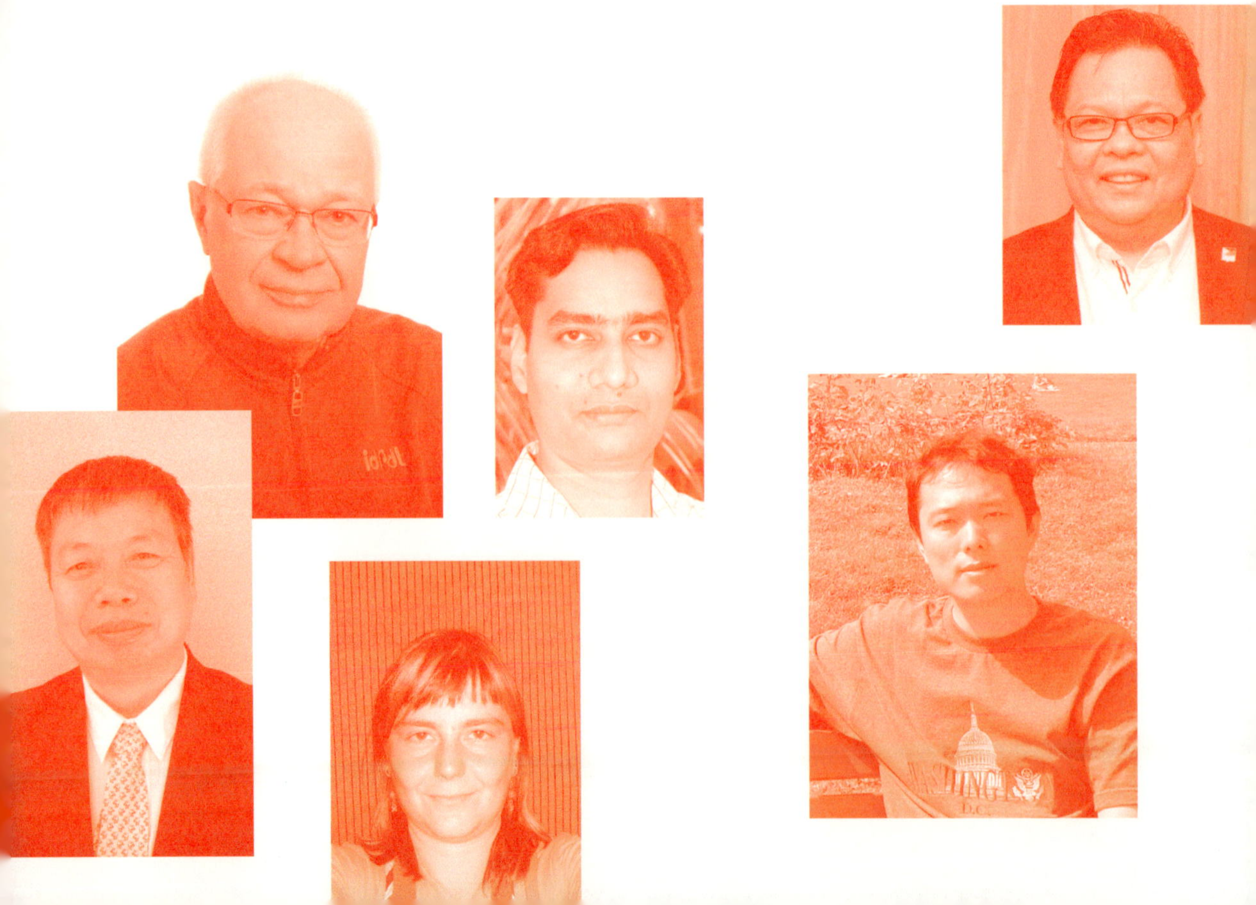

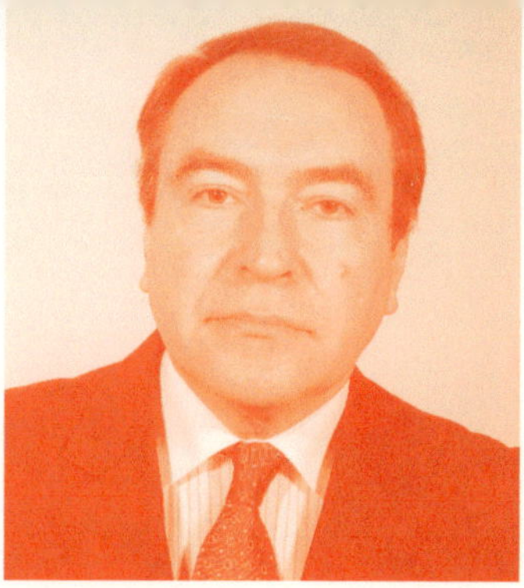
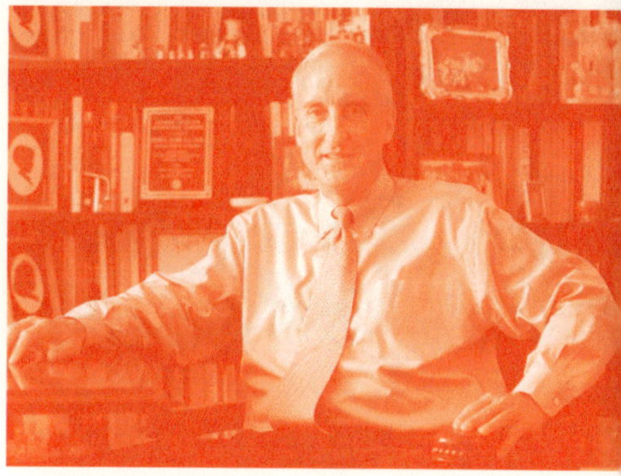
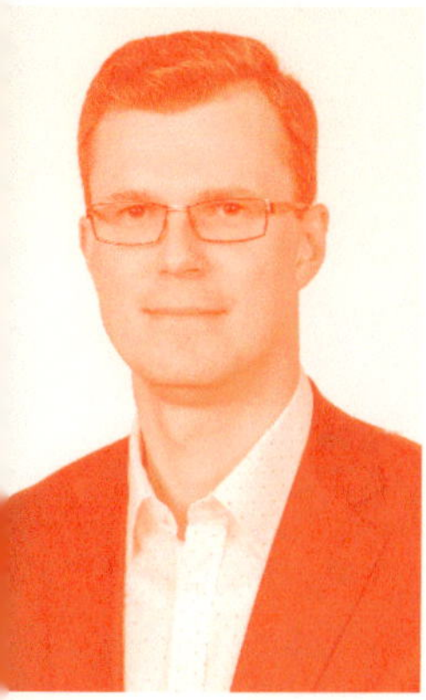
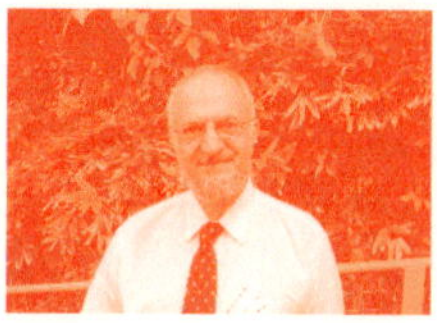
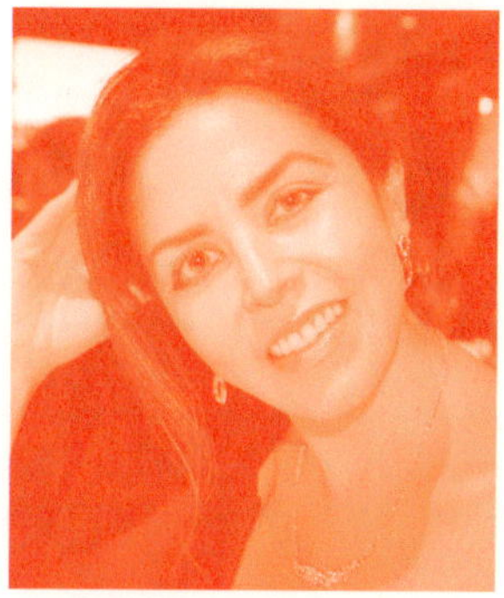

Supporting open minds since 2005

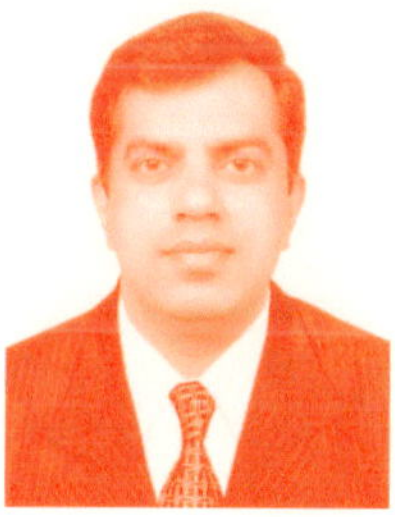
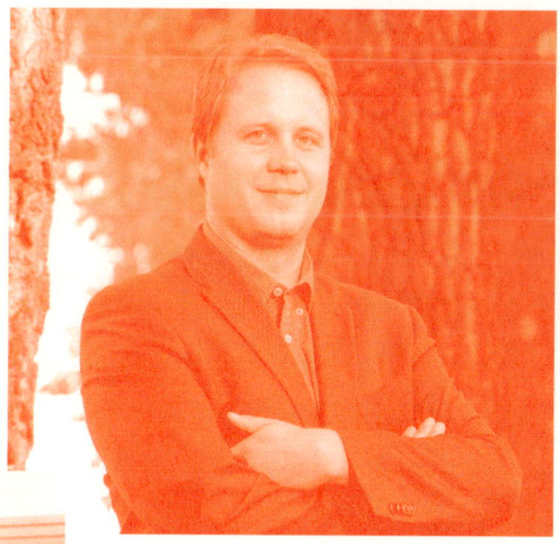
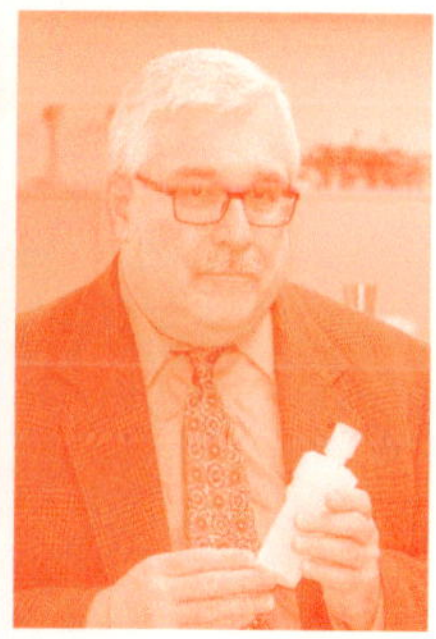
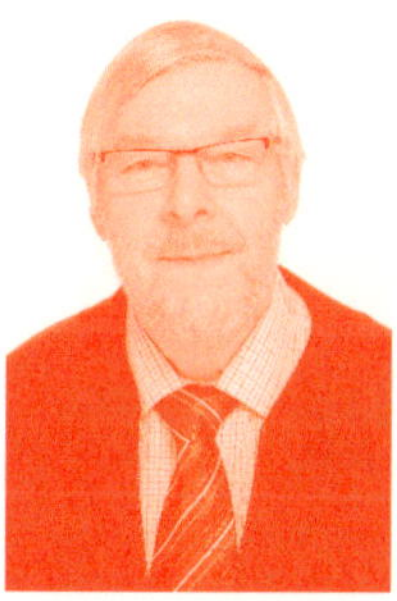
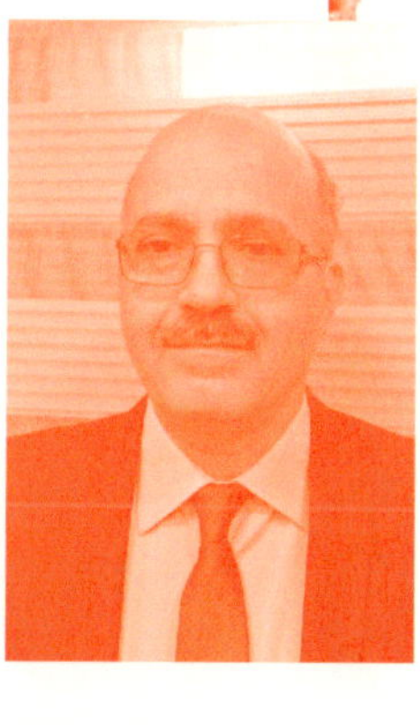
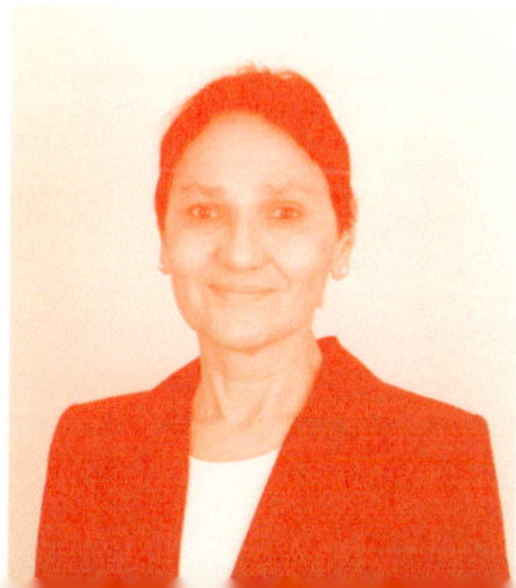
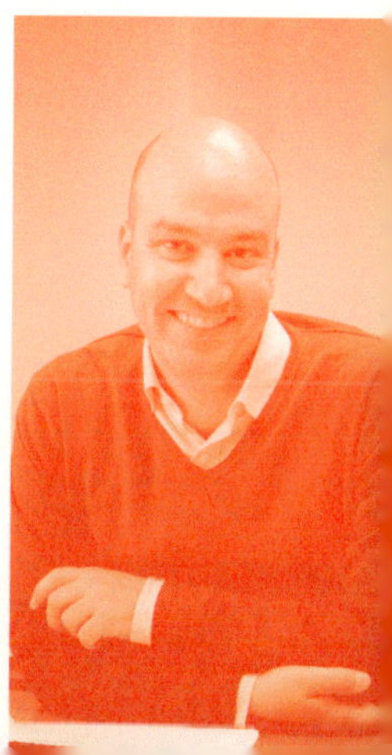

Tibia Pathology and Fractures
http://dx.doi.org/10.5772/intechopen.87317
Edited by Dimitrios D. Nikolopoulos, George K. Safos and John Michos

Contributors
Sabah S. Moshref, Yasir S. Jamal, Amro M. Al-Hibshi, Abdullah M. Mohammed Kaki, Reiner Wirbel, Luis Bahamonde, Alvaro Zamorano, Pierluca Zecchetto, Konstantinos Ditsios, Triantafyllos Katsimentzas, Tryfon Ditsios, John Thomas Riehl, Jan Szatkowski, Christian M. Schmidt II, Tahsin Beyzadeoglu, Kerem Yildirim, Tuna Pehlivanoglu

First published in London, United Kingdom, 2020 by IntechOpen
IntechOpen is the global imprint of INTECHOPEN LIMITED, registered in England and Wales, registration number: 11086078, 7th floor, 10 Lower Thames Street, London, EC3R 6AF, United Kingdom
Printed in Croatia

British Library Cataloguing-in-Publication Data
A catalogue record for this book is available from the British Library

Additional hard and PDF copies can be obtained from orders@intechopen.com

Tibia Pathology and Fractures
Edited by Dimitrios D. Nikolopoulos, George K. Safos and John Michos
p. cm.
Print ISBN 978-1-83962-406-3
Online ISBN 978-1-83962-407-0
eBook (PDF) ISBN 978-1-83962-408-7

For EU product safety concerns:
IN TECH d.o.o., Prolaz Marije Krucifikse Kozulić 3, 51000 Rijeka, Croatia, info@intechopen.com or visit our website at intechopen.com.

Meet the editors

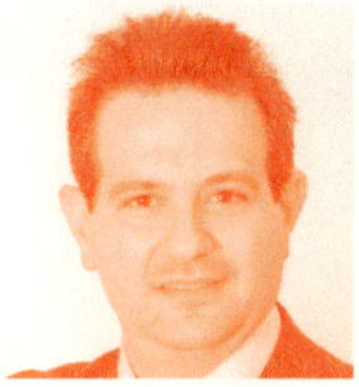

Dr. Dimitrios D. Nikolopoulos (MD, PhD) is a sports medicine-specialized orthopedic surgeon and arthroscopist. He focuses on sports injuries and mainly in shoulder, hip, knee, foot, and ankle pathology. He has performed arthroscopic restoration of hip, knee, and ankle cartilage, as well as treatment and surgical correction of foot disorders. He has published 42 original scientific articles in prestigious scientific journals in the United States, Europe, and Greece referring to knee (valgus knee) and shoulder (arthroscopic and minimally invasive new techniques) surgery, osteoporotic spine and hip fractures, and research into the in vitro environment of bone and cartilage metabolism. He has more than 180 citations in research projects on valgus knee and cartilage ankle restoration. He has also presented over 180 oral and poster presentations internationally.

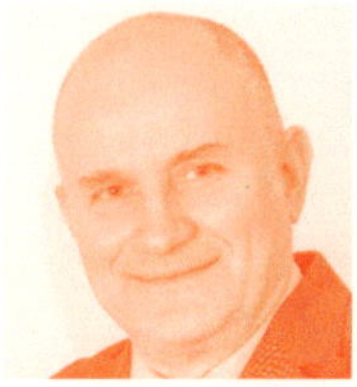

Dr. George K. Safos (MD) specializes in orthopedic surgery and traumatology with interest in sports medicine (knee, hip, ankle, elbow, and shoulder arthroscopic surgery) as well as total hip and knee replacement surgery. As a well-published doctor, he now serves as a medical orthopedic consultant and primary doctor to various athletic teams, dance groups, as well as foreign diplomatic missions. He is a graduate of Athens University Medical School and completed his residency in orthopedic surgery and traumatology at the General Hospital of Asklepeion Voulas. He then completed two fellowships in the United States, namely at the National Institutes of Health (NIH) in Bethesda, Maryland, as well as at the University of Miami-Orthopedic Department. A postgraduate degree in Tissue Banking at the National University of Singapore with a United Nations scholarship soon followed.

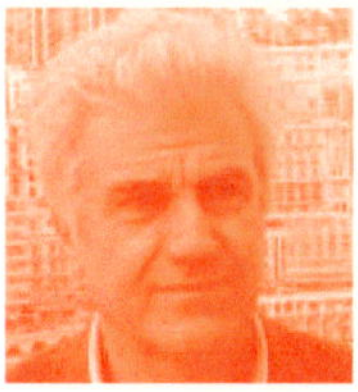

Dr. John Michos has been Director of the 4th Orthopaedic Department in Asklepion Voulas Hospital since 2004. He studied in Athens University Medical School and qualified as an orthopedic surgeon in 1985. He worked in UK hospitals from 1985 to 1989 and thereafter in the Asklepion Voulas Hospital in Athens. His special interest is knee surgery, including arthroplasty and ligament reconstruction surgery. He established the Sports Medicine Clinic of Asklepion Voulas Hospital. He also served as President of the Hellenic Orthopaedic Association in 2011.

Contents

Preface

The tibia is the long bone located in the lower leg between the knee and foot. Tibial fractures are common and usually caused by an injury or repetitive strain on the bone. The severity and type of fracture may vary and needs immediate therapy—usually operative—especially the intraarticular fractures of the knee or the ankle (plateau or platform fractures). Variation on the anatomical or mechanical axis of the tibia may cause knee or ankle arthritis in the middle or long follow-up period. Open reduction and internal fixation are the gold standard for proximal or distal tibial fractures, whereas conservative (injections) or surgical (high tibia osteotomy) therapies also offer primary arthritic changes before joint replacement.

Dr. Dimitrios D. Nikolopoulos
President of Foundation of Orthopaedic Research and Training,
Central Clinic of Athens,
Greece

Dr. George K. Safos (MD)
Central Clinic of Athens,
Greece

Dr. John Michos (MD, PhD)
Director of 4th Orthopaedic Clinic of Asklepion Voulas Hospital,
Greece

Section 1

Intra-Articular Tibia Fractures

Chapter 1

Tibial Plateau Fracture

Christian M. Schmidt II, Jan P. Szatkowski and John T. Riehl

Abstract

Tibial plateau fractures are a common orthopedic injury. These fractures involve the articular surface of the tibia that is part of the knee joint. Plateau fractures can range from low energy injuries with little or no displacement to complex fractures with significant associated injuries. Stability of these injuries depends on a combination of bony and associated ligamentous injuries. Treatment consists of a wide spectrum of therapies which have been discussed in this chapter. Complications such as compartment syndrome, post-traumatic arthritis, chronic pain, malunion, and wound problems (in addition to other complications) can develop.

Keywords: Tibial plateau, fracture, Schatzker, buttress plate, Bicondylar, calcium phosphate cement

1. Introduction

Fractures involving the tibial articular surface account for a little over 1% of all long bone fractures, 56.9% of all proximal tibia fractures/dislocations, and 8% of all fractures in the elderly [1–4]. They have an annual incidence of 10.3 per 100,000 [5]. The combined incidence of a patient having a tibial plateau fracture with associated polytrauma on admission has been estimated at 16–40% [6–8]. The age distribution is bimodal for both males and females which is similar to what is seen in other periarticular injuries [1]. The majority of fractures occur in males (70%) with men aged 40–44 years being the most affected patient population overall [4, 5]. Comminuted fractures are more common in males [3]. The highest incidence for tibial plateau fractures in females occurs between age 55 and 59 [4]. There is a shift of incidence between males and females that occurs after the age of 60 with females predominating (61%) [4, 9]. With an increase in life expectancy as well as a large aging population in many developed countries it is expected that the incidence of low-energy tibial plateau fractures will continue to increase.

2. Injury mechanism

The injury mechanism seen in tibial plateau fractures is largely age-dependent. The majority of tibial plateau fractures in the elderly are due to low energy falls. With an aging population and associated osteoporosis, the incidence of this injury is increasing. Osteopenia and osteoporosis play a large role in the fracture mechanisms and patterns observed. In the elderly, lateral fracture patterns are seen more commonly than medial. The forces acting on the bone in conjunction with the bone quality determine the resulting fracture patterns [10]. Bone quality influences fracture patterns with low bone density decreasing the force necessary for injury. A higher incidence of compression fracture patterns tends to be seen in such cases despite lower energy injury mechanisms. In the younger population, high energy mechanisms predominate. Male gender is more common. The injury mechanism can involve motor vehicles, sports, and falls from height. The most common mechanism of injury overall is pedestrian struck by motorized vehicles (30%) and the second most common is low energy falls (22%) [11].

The magnitude and direction of the force of injury many times will influence the fracture pattern. Angular, axial, and compression forces can all lead to failure of the condyles. Axial load is usually a predominant component of the injury mechanism and produces higher energy at failure than angular forces. In general, greater axial load results in more severe fractures with increased comminution, fragment displacement, and associated soft tissue injury. In a cadaver study [12] that looked at mechanisms of injury it was found that pure valgus forces resulted in the typical lateral split fractures, axial forces resulted in joint compression fractures, and a combination of axial and valgus forces resulted in split depression fractures. The same study also concluded that an intact MCL is required for an isolated lateral plateau fracture to occur because the MCL acts as the pivot point causing the lateral femoral condyle to impact the lateral tibial plateau. The proximal tibia is more readily subject to valgus force because of an anatomic predisposition with 5–7° of knee valgus in normal anatomic alignment and due to lateral side impacts being a more common injury mechanism.

3. Anatomy

The superior tibia widens from the diaphysis proximally (**Figure 1**). The proximal anterior tibia forms the tibial tubercle and provides the attachment of the patellar tendon. Lateral to the tibial tubercle is Gerdy's tubercle which serves as the insertion site of the distal iliotibial band. The lateral proximal tibia forms the lateral tibial condyle and the inferior aspect of this serves as the attachment site of the anterior compartment muscles of the leg. The origin of the anterior muscles must be elevated in order to place an anterolateral plate. Medially and proximal to the tibial tubercle is the medial condyle. The medial condyle is less often involved in failure than the lateral condyle. The palpable fibular head (which is extra-articular to the knee joint) is found posterolateral and serves as the attachment site of the fibular collateral ligament and the biceps femoris tendon. The peroneal nerve wraps from posterior to anterior around the neck of the fibula. Even though the fibula does not participate in the knee joint articulation it does act as a buttress for the lateral tibial plateau. Because of this, associated proximal fibular fractures can result in greater valgus instability.

The medial and lateral tibial plateaus articulate directly with the medial and lateral condyles of the femur. The tibial articular width is slightly wider than the femoral articular width (tibia:femur articular width ratio was found to be 1.01 ± 0.04 in one study of healthy knees) [13]. With this in mind it might be useful to use the femur as a reference to judge pathologic tibial plateau widening and adequacy of intraoperative reductions [13, 14]. The lateral plateau is more proximal and slightly convex whereas the medial plateau is more concave and slightly distal to the lateral plateau. The medial plateau bears around 60% of the total load borne across the knee. Relative to the tibial diaphysis, the plateau is slightly varus due to the proximal nature of the lateral tibial condyle [15]. The concavity of the medial plateau allows for greater congruity of the medial tibia with the femoral condyle compared to the lateral. The tibial plateau slopes about 15° posteroinferiorly making

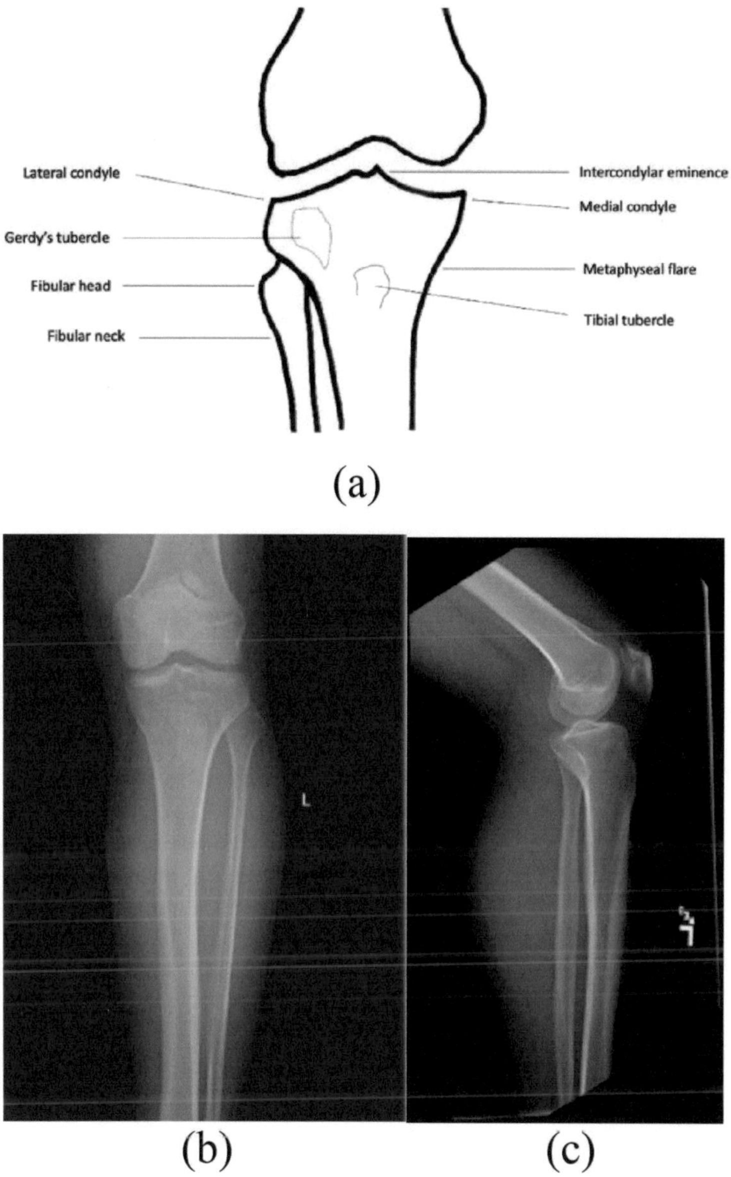

Figure 1.
Proximal tibia anatomy (A) and normal plain radiographs of the tibial plateau anterior-posterior (AP) view (B) and lateral view (C) (Drawing and radiographs: courtesy of John Riehl MD & www.johnriehl.com).

the anterior plateau proximal and posterior plateau more distal [16]. The medial plateau's posterior tibial slope is greater than the lateral plateau's posterior slope [17]. Variations to an individual's normal coronal and sagittal alignment can be crucial for surgical planning, so side by side knee radiographs can be useful in assessing each patient's anatomical variation [15]. The tibial plateau surfaces are covered by articular hyaline cartilage and partially by menisci composed of fibrocartilage. The lateral plateau is more covered by its meniscus than the medial plateau is. The intercondylar eminence consists of two spines, one medial and one lateral. The intercondylar eminence is non-articular and splits the proximal tibia into the lateral and medial plateaus. The medial spine serves as the attachment site of the anterior cruciate ligament and the posterior cruciate ligament attaches posteriorly on the proximal tibia.

4. Classification

Fracture classifications are widely used in clinical practice in order to help communicate and plan treatment as well as to aid in prognosis and to provide standards for clinical research. Commonly used classifications include the Schatzker, Hohl-Moore, Luo, and Orthopedic Trauma Association classifications.

4.1 Schatzker classification

The Schatzker Classification (**Figure 2**) was first published in 1979 and is one of the most commonly used tibial plateau fracture classifications still today [18]. The system divides tibial plateau fractures into six types designated from I to VI. The main limitation of this classification system is its failure to account for many important tibial plateau fracture patterns [19–23]. The Schatzker classification was based on the use of AP plain radiographs of the knee and because of this it is primarily beneficial in analysis of sagittal fracture lines on the medial and lateral plateaus leaving out fractures in the coronal plane.

Type I fractures are pure split fractures. The lateral femoral condyle is driven into the lateral tibial plateau resulting in a sagittal fracture line that splits the lateral tibial plateau with a fracture line running laterally and inferiorly creating a wedge-shaped fragment. There is no associated articular depression or crush. These fractures are most commonly seen in young patients with healthy bone. Percutaneous screw fixation and lateral buttress plate fixation are two surgical treatments commonly employed for these fractures.

Type II fractures are split fractures combined with articular depression. These are similar to type I fractures with a lateral split except there is also lateral articular surface depression. The injury mechanism in type II fractures is typically either high energy, low energy with poor bone quality, or both high energy and poor bone quality.

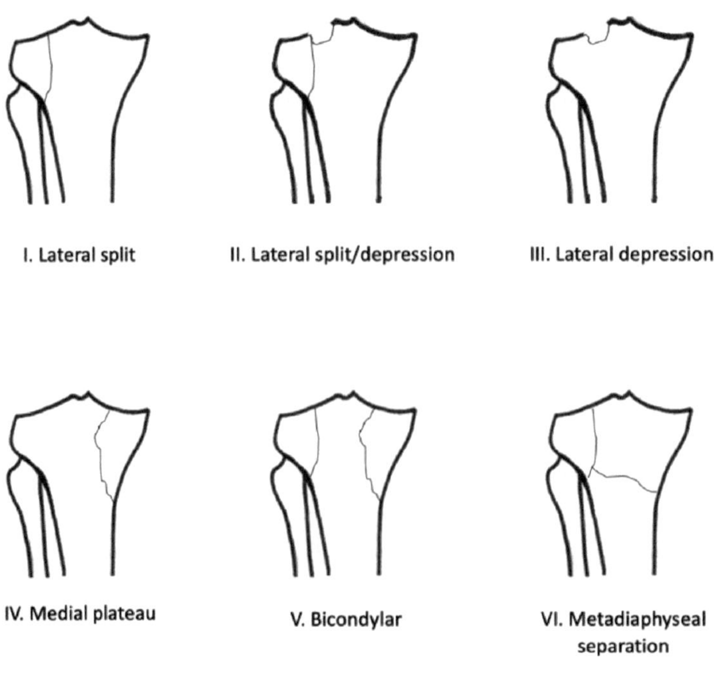

Figure 2.
Schatzker classification of tibial plateau fractures (Drawings created by www.johnriehl.com).

Treatment is dictated by the degree of joint depression, width of condylar split, and knee stability. Many Schatzker type II fractures are treated surgically with the elevation of the articular depression with some sort of bone grafting or graft substitute. The fracture is then often stabilized with articular surface compression and lateral buttress plating. Newer locking plates have shown promise in maintaining articular reduction following compression, especially in patients with poor bone quality.

Type III fractures are pure depression fractures. They do not have a lateral split as seen in type I and II. This is most commonly seen in elderly patients with poor subchondral bone quality from osteopenia or osteoporosis. The femoral condyle presses into the lateral tibial plateau resulting in depression of the articular surface rather than a split because of the underlying poor bone quality. The surgical treatment of these fractures involves elevating and supporting the articular surface.

Type IV fractures are medial condylar fractures (**Figure 3**). Schatzker describes these with two subtypes. In these subtypes, the medial plateau is either split off as a wedge fragment or depressed and comminuted. Either of these subtypes can also include fractures of the tibial spine. Pure medial tibial plateau fractures are rare. Fracture lines usually include the tibial spine and on occasion the lateral plateau. This fracture is more commonly associated with a higher energy mechanism of injury and results in a loss of medial buttressing. Non-operative management will often result in varus deformity. Medial tibial plateau fracture types are considered to be variants of knee dislocations. The ACL and MCL are intact but the lateral plateau and tibial shaft shift laterally away from the medial fragment. This puts patients at higher risk for neurovascular injury and compartment syndrome [24, 25]. The incidence of compartment syndrome may be as high as 53% in this fracture pattern [25].

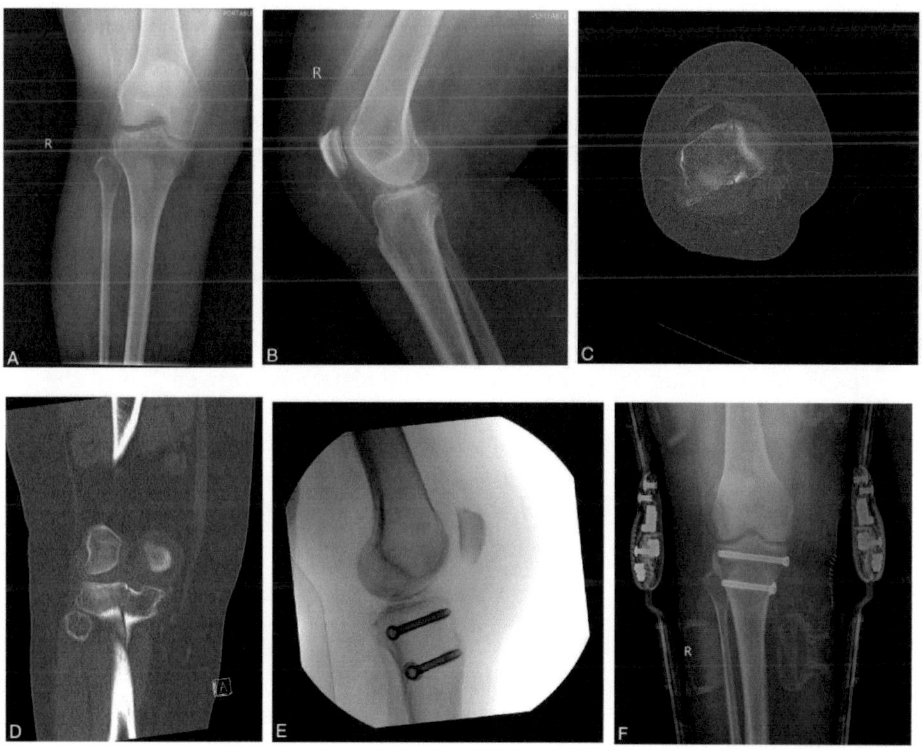

Figure 3.
Patient with multitrauma and a Schatzker IV fracture seen on plain radiographs (A and B) and CT scan (C and D) fixed with compression screws (E and F) (Radiographs and intraoperative imaging courtesy of John Riehl MD).

Type V fractures are bicondylar fractures. In this fracture pattern, both medial and lateral tibial plateaus are fractured. A portion of the metaphysis and diaphysis remain continuous, however, differentiating it from a type VI pattern. Schatzker IV-VI fractures are most often the result of a high energy mechanism of injury. Surgical treatment (when indicated) for type V fractures includes reduction and fixation of both condyles in order to reestablish stability, which is often done with dual approaches and dual plating, but may be done occasionally through a single approach with locked plating depending on the fracture pattern and displacement.

Type VI fractures are tibial plateau fractures with dissociation of the metaphysis and diaphysis. The hallmark of these fractures is either a horizontal or oblique fracture line that separates the diaphysis from the joint segment. These fractures are very unstable. Reduction and fixation of both plateaus is often necessary. These patients are at increased risk for neurovascular and soft tissue compromise [26–28]. The literature reports an incidence of 17–34% of compartment syndrome in this fracture pattern [25, 26, 29].

4.2 Hohl-Moore classification

The Hohl-Moore classification (**Figure 4**) was developed in 1981 and reevaluated in 1987 based on 988 tibial plateau fractures seen at University of Southern California from 1970 to 1979 [2, 30]. It has been used to classify fracture-dislocations not described completely by the Schatzker classification which accounts for around 10% of all tibial plateau fractures. These fracture patterns more commonly involve the lateral plateau (79%) and are more associated with instability, soft tissue injury, vascular compromise, and compartment syndrome [2].

Type I fractures are coronal split fractures. These are found in 37% of tibial plateau fracture-dislocation [30]. These injuries are more clearly seen on lateral radiographs. They usually involve the medial plateau and the oblique fracture runs in a coronal-transverse plane. Common associations include avulsion fractures of the fibula or Gerdy's tubercle and capsular disruptions. Treatment of this fracture ranges from nonoperative casting to percutaneous screw fixation or ORIF with plate fixation. Treatment depends on the stability of the knee and the extent of the tibial plateau the fracture involves.

Type II fractures are entire condylar fractures. Either the entire medial or more commonly the lateral condyle is fractured. The fracture line extends beyond the tibial spine into the opposite plateau differentiating it from a traditional Schatzker I or IV. Soft tissue injury occurs in many of these patients. Opposite compartment collateral ligament injury occurs in up to 50% of patients and neurovascular injury in 12% [30]. Treatments range again depending on stability and extent of articular involvement.

Type III are rim avulsion fractures. The lateral plateau is involved 93% of the time but the medial plateau can be involved as well [2]. Tearing of the ACL or PCL or both is commonly seen. Neurovascular injury is common in this fracture pattern occurring up to 30% of the time [30]. Instability is generally present and usually requires fixation. Soft tissue repair or reconstruction is considered.

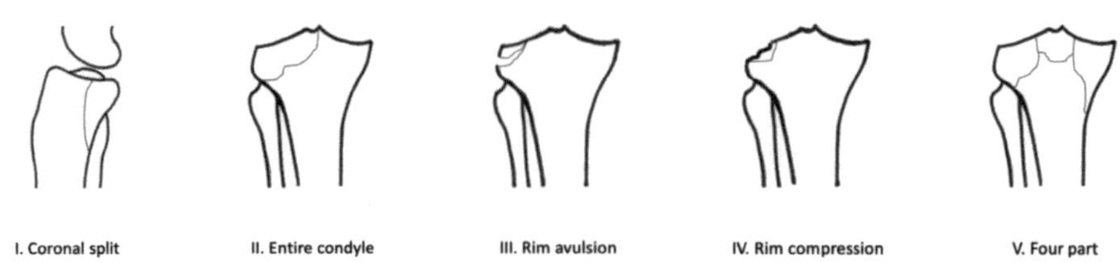

Figure 4.
Hohl-Moore classification of tibial plateau fractures (Drawings created by www.johnriehl.com).

Type IV are rim compression fractures. This fracture accounts for 12% of all tibial plateau fracture-dislocations [30]. The lateral plateau is much more commonly involved [2]. Collateral ligament injury of the unfractured condyle commonly occurs and cruciate ligament injury occurs in more than 75% of cases [30].

Type V are four-part fractures. These account for 10% of all fracture dislocations [30]. The medial and lateral condyles of the tibia are fractured as well as the intercondylar eminence. These fractures are highly unstable due to loss of the stabilizing effects of the collateral and cruciate ligaments. Neurovascular injury occurs as high as 50% of the time [30]. With their severe instability, these fractures will usually require surgical management.

4.3 AO/OTA

The AO/OTA classification system is a more comprehensive classification system that was first published in 1996 with the intent of bringing uniformity to all fracture classification [31]. This fracture classification uses two main components, fracture location and morphology. Localization defines the specific bone and the segment of bone involved (proximal, distal, shaft). Morphology classifies the fracture type, group, and subgroup delineating articular involvement and simple vs. multifragmentary patterns. With tibial plateau fractures the localization number is 41 (4 is for the tibia and 1 is for the proximal segment). Morphology types include extra-articular, partial articular and complete articular fractures which are labeled A, B, and C respectively and then fractures are further grouped and subgrouped using numbers 1–3 and 0.1–0.3 further specifying the fractures specific morphology. The AO/OTA system subcategories by degree of comminution of the metaphysis and articular surface making it more comprehensive than the Schatzker Classification and able to distinguish ranges of severity of high energy patterns.

4.4 Luo three-column classification

The Luo Three-Column Classification (**Figure 5**) was published in 2010 based on 3D conceptualization of the tibial plateau and is useful in describing multiplanar complex tibial plateau fractures [19–21]. Traditionally the treatment

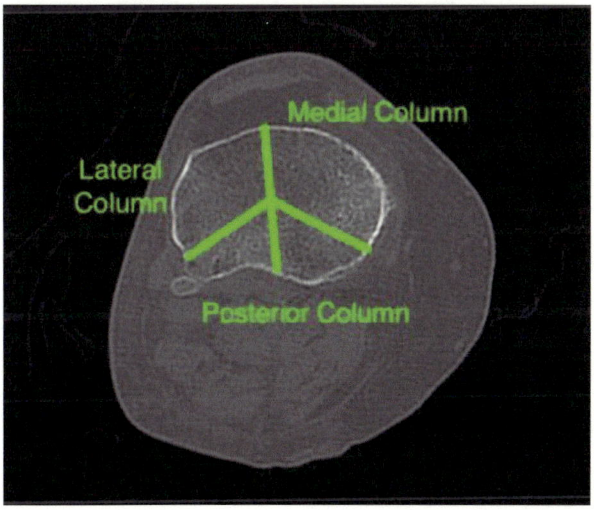

Figure 5.
Luo Three Column Classification (Radiograph courtesy of John Riehl MD).

and classification of tibial plateau fractures was based on two-dimensional classification systems like Moore and Schatzker that used plain radiographs whereas Luo uses axial CT scan images. Luo divides the tibial plateau using three intersecting lines dividing the plateau into three columns (medial, lateral, and posterior). The meeting point is the middle of the two tibial spines. The anterior line connects the midpoint of the plateau to the tibial tuberosity. The medial line travels from the midpoint to the posteromedial ridge and the lateral line is drawn from the midpoint to just anterior to the fibular head. Fractures can be defined as zero, one, two, or three column fractures. With this classification a column is considered fractured only if a cortical split is present in the column, thus a pure depression fracture (Schatzker III) is considered a zero column fracture. This classification system is useful in preoperative planning especially when there is posterior involvement. The posterior segment has been shown to be more prevalent than previously recognized and failure to identify and manage it has been associated with misalignment and functional instability [22, 32, 33].

5. Clinical evaluation

5.1 History

It is important to obtain a thorough history in all tibial plateau fractures. The mechanism of injury should be assessed to give an idea of the severity of the injury and the need for urgent or emergent management. Low energy falls or twisting injuries are more likely to have a lower risk of neurovascular injury or compartment syndrome whereas falls from a height, motor vehicle accidents, and pedestrians struck by a vehicle are more likely to be higher risk and may necessitate more urgent or emergent management. Although knowing the mechanism of injury can be helpful, the fracture pattern is also extremely important in determining the treatment approach and risk for complications. Location and severity of pain, the timing of the injury, associated injuries, and any treatments administered are helpful pieces of information. Past medical history should be assessed for tobacco use, prior knee problems, ambulatory status prior to injury, and medical comorbidities (such as pulmonary disease, diabetes, vascular disease, cancers, renal disease, nutritional deficiencies, previous poor DEXA scan results, as well as use of immunosuppressive medicines). Medical comorbidities and certain medications can affect bone quality, increase risk for postoperative infection, and inhibit wound healing. The patient's activity level, social support, mental condition, and employment status should be known in order to make an appropriate surgical and rehabilitation plan.

5.2 Physical exam

As a part of the initial assessment of tibial plateau fractures, the physical exam should attempt to rule out soft tissue compromise, open fractures, compartment syndrome, and neurovascular injury. A circumferential assessment of the overlying skin and a neurovascular baseline status should be conducted. Circumferential skin and soft tissue inspection and palpation should be done to assess for open injury and severity of soft tissue injury. The severity of soft tissue injury may be further defined based on size, character, and location of swelling, contusions, and fracture blisters. Soft tissue assessment is key to determining surgical approaches and timing.

A non-compressible, firm extremity and pain with passive stretching are suggestive of compartment syndrome. Compartment syndrome should be monitored for throughout the patient's stay since this can develop days after injury or surgery. Measurement of compartment pressures in high energy fracture patterns or unresponsive patients may be beneficial on presentation and may need to be repeated based on clinical assessment. If the diagnosis is made in conjunction with elevated compartment pressures or if the diagnosis is clear on the physical exam, a fasciotomy will need to be performed.

For high-energy injuries especially (such as fracture-dislocations and metaphyseal-diaphyseal dissociation patterns) it is imperative to obtain a thorough neurovascular assessment. Vascular injury is rare overall but delays >8 h in diagnosis and surgical intervention can result in lower extremity amputation rates as high as 86% [34–36]. Neurovascular assessment should include testing for sensation patterns in the distribution of tibial, superficial peroneal, saphenous, and sural nerves as well as extremity color and temperature, capillary refill, and distal pulses including the posterior tibial and dorsalis pedis. Results should be compared with the contralateral side. Any differences in pulses or sensation can be further investigated with an ankle-brachial index (ABI) measurement. For some high-energy fractures, consideration may be given to obtain ABI regardless. An ABI > 0.8 has a remarkably high negative predictive value, approaching 100%. With ABI <0.9 further vascular assessment with a CT arteriogram and/or a vascular surgery consultation should be obtained [34].

Varus and valgus stress testing may be necessary to assess for instability if this is unclear based on radiographic assessment. Valgus instability is important in determining indications for surgical management, especially in lateral tibial plateau fractures. If instability is present it may not resolve without surgical fracture reduction and fixation [37, 38].

6. Radiology (plain radiographs, stress views, CT, MRI)

Imaging is a large part of the surgical planning process. The imaging modalities used range from plain radiographs to CT with 3D reconstruction and MRI.

6.1 Plain radiographs

The diagnosis of a tibial plateau fractures is usually made initially by plain radiographs. For some simple fractures, this may be the only imaging modality necessary. Typically anteroposterior (AP) and lateral views of the knee are obtained for plain radiograph assessment. An additional view, the caudal view (also known as the "tibial plateau view") is shot 10–15° caudally from a typical 90° AP view and is used to provide a view in line with the plane of the plateau. This is done to account for the 15° posteroinferior slope of the plateau surface. In this view, the proximal articular surface can be viewed as a single radiodense line which allows better assessment than lateral and AP views of articular depression [16]. Radiographs of the entire tibia should be obtained as well. Oblique views have also been used to assess the fracture lines and degree of displacement, however, they are not routine now that computed tomography (CT) scans have largely filled the need that was once provided by additional views. Of note, it has been shown that plain radiographs alone can miss insufficiency fractures in osteopenic patients [39].

Traction radiographs are helpful when there is substantial displacement to better assess the fracture anatomy in both plain radiographs and CT scans. This can be obtained by manual traction or spanning external fixators.

Contralateral radiographs may be helpful in severely comminuted fractures to serve as a template for reduction, condylar width, coronal alignment, and the posterior slope of the plateau in the sagittal plane.

6.2 Computed tomography (CT)

Computed tomography (CT) scans have become a routine part of the assessment of tibial plateau fractures (**Figure 6**). Axial CT cuts are especially helpful in visualizing posteromedial fracture lines (**Figure** 7). Axial CT and reconstructions provide important insight into fracture anatomy as well as serving as an aid in preoperative planning. It has been demonstrated in numerous studies that the use of CT scans allows surgeons to more reliably classify fractures which aids in providing the most appropriate treatment formulation [40–46]. CT allows accurate visualization of articular displacement and comminution more readily than what is observed with plain radiographs [46]. CT also allows for better assessment of location and orientation of fracture lines as well as the degree of depression and size of articular segments, which provides important information in preoperative planning.

6.3 Magnetic resonance imaging (MRI)

Magnetic resonance imaging (MRI) continues to gain wider acceptance in use for evaluation of tibial plateau fractures. Some argue it is indicated to adequately assess and treat soft tissue injuries especially in fractures due to high energy mechanisms which have a high percentage of ligamentous and meniscal pathology [47]. MRI is more sensitive than CT in detecting ligamentous and meniscal injuries which are both common occurrences in tibial plateau fractures [48]. MRI is the gold standard when it comes to detecting occult fractures not seen on plain radiograph.

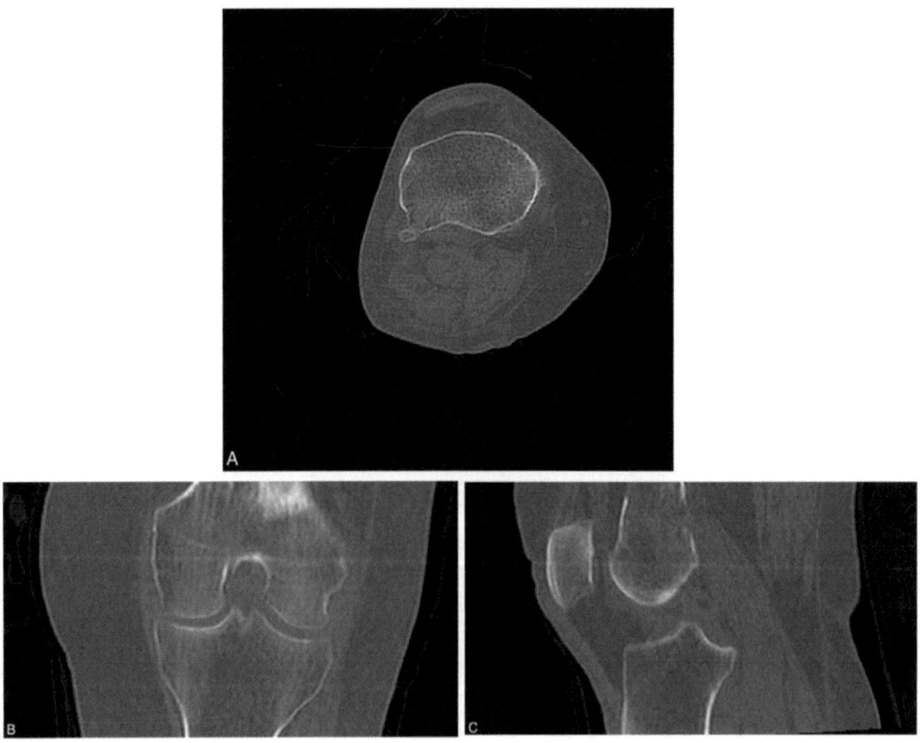

Figure 6.
CT of a normal tibial plateau axial view (A), coronal view (B), and Sagittal view (C) (Images courtesy of John Riehl MD).

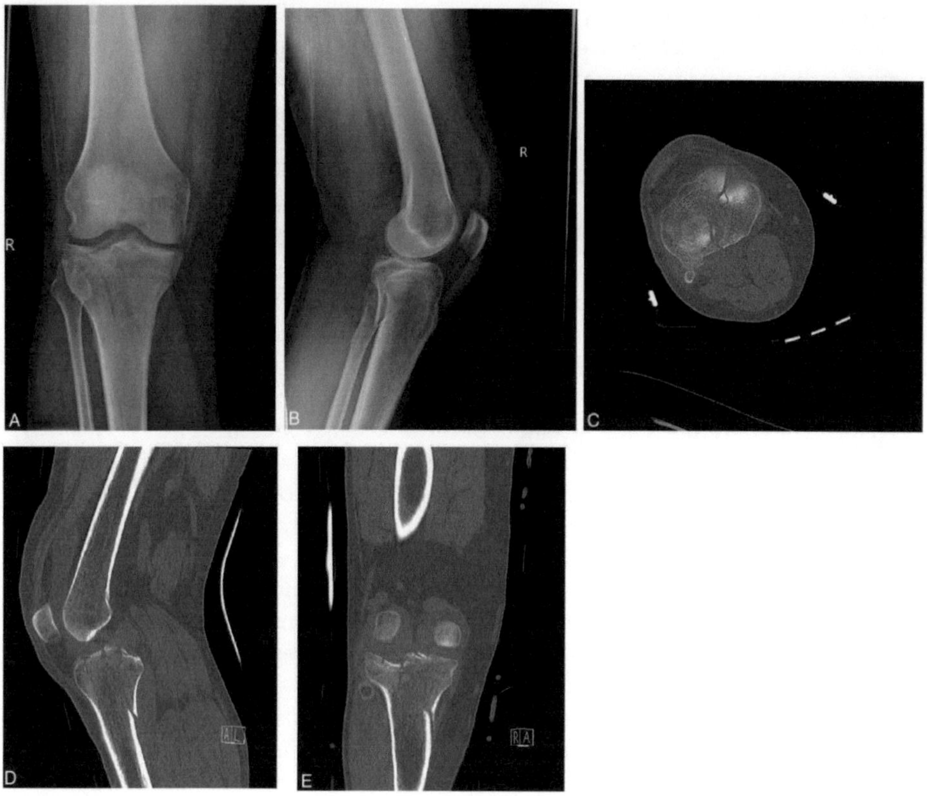

Figure 7.
CT allows for better visualization and more accurate classification compared with plain radiographs (A,B) of this bicondylar tibial plateau fracture more clearly seen in the axial view (C), sagittal view (D), and coronal view (E) (Images courtesy of John Riehl MD).

7. Compartment syndrome

Compartment syndrome (CS) is a serious complication of trauma and other conditions that cause bleeding, edema or vascular compromise. Progressive swelling of a limb increases mass within the myofascial compartment due to accumulation of blood or fluid as well as inflammation. The inelasticity of the muscle fascia and connective tissue results in increased pressure in the compartment compressing thin-walled veins leading to venous hypertension and tissue ischemia. Compartment pressure increases further once cellular death accelerates and lysis of cells releases osmotically active fluid into the interstitial space. Myonecrosis may occur within 2 h of injury [49] and after 6–8 h irreversible nerve damage occurs.

CS can be quite common in certain patterns of tibial plateau fractures, and has been found to be as high as 53% in Schatzker type IV fractures [25]. Overall the reported incidence of CS following tibial plateau fracture ranges from 0.7 to 12% [26, 29, 50–53]. Although a somewhat controversial topic with conflicting findings in the literature, acute compartment syndrome requiring fasciotomy has been reported in some studies to significantly increase the rate of non-unions [27] and infections [27, 54–56]. On the other hand, Ruffalo et al. [57] found no increase in the association of nonunion and infection. In medial plateau fractures, one study found a 67% CS rate when the fracture entered the joint line lateral to the tibial spine and exited through the medial metaphysis, 33% CS rate when the fracture is within the spine and 14% when the fracture is medial to the intercondylar spine [24]. CS was found to have a higher incidence in Schatzker type IV (53%) compared with type VI (18%) fracture patterns [25]. However, this result was not consistent throughout the literature, and another group reported compartment syndrome to be relatively rare in type IV and only type VI patterns were significantly more likely to develop it [26]. CS was least common in Schatzker type I and II fractures [26]. The two biggest radiographic predictors of CS were fracture length and fibular head fracture [26, 28].

Early diagnosis of CS is crucial for avoiding the substantial morbidity caused by its late sequelae. A clinical diagnosis of CS can be difficult to make even when the generally accepted clinical signs of CS are present, which include worsening pain that is out of proportion to the clinical situation, pain with passive stretch, and paresthesia/hypoesthesia. These clinical signs and symptoms have been shown to have low sensitivity [58, 59]. Also, clinical findings can be difficult to obtain in polytrauma patients and impossible to assess in sedated patients. Late diagnosis can be diminished by frequent or continuous measurement of intramuscular pressure (IMP). When to initiate IMP monitoring is still controversial but whenever clinical examination is unreliable in an at-risk patient measurement of IMP could be considered. When using IMP, diastolic differential pressure (delta p) <30 mm Hg has been used as a threshold for compartment syndrome requiring fasciotomy. Prayson et al. [60] warn against using a single measurement <30 mm Hg alone as this may not be clinically significant. In their series they found that this can occur transiently in patients without evidence of compartment syndrome. About 84% of their lower extremity fracture patients had at least one delta p < 30 mm Hg and 58% had a delta p < 20 mm Hg. Instead, McQueen et al. [61] suggest a threshold for fasciotomy of an IMP<30 mm Hg for two consecutive hours or more, which had a sensitivity for diagnosis of CS of 94%.

One of the potential pitfalls of using pressure measurements is that intraoperative diastolic blood pressure measurements have been shown by Tornetta et al. [62] to give spuriously low delta p values and lead to unnecessary fasciotomies. The authors of this study recommend use of preoperative blood pressure values when calculating delta p in patients under general anesthesia unless the patient is to remain under anesthesia for numerous hours. IMP values also vary with proximity to the fracture site and muscular depth. Pressures are highest when measuring within 5 cm of the fracture [63] and centrally in the muscle [64]. Most recommend obtaining the measurement within 5 cm of the fracture site but the standarizability of this is still controversial.

8. Associated soft tissue injuries

Soft tissue injuries occur commonly in tibial plateau fractures. Overall soft tissue injury incidence has been estimated between 73 and 99% from MRI studies [65–67]. In an MRI analysis of 103 operative tibial plateau fracture patients, Gardner et al. [65] only found 1 patient who had complete absence of soft tissue injury. Collateral or cruciate injuries were sustained in 77% of patients and lateral and medial meniscus pathology was seen in 91% and 44%, respectively. Similar results were seen in a study on nonoperative tibial plateau fracture patients with 90% having significant soft tissue injuries, 80% with meniscal tears and 40% with ligament disruptions [66].

8.1 Ligament injury

Overall ligamentous injury incidence has been estimated by MRI studies to be between 40 and 77% [47, 65, 66]. MRI studies in the literature estimate that complete anterior cruciate ligament (ACL) tears have an incidence of 11–44%, posterior cruciate ligament (PCL) 8–40%, lateral collateral ligament (LCL) 29%, medial collateral ligament (MCL) 32%, and posterolateral corner (PLC) injuries 45–68% [47, 65]. Higher energy fracture (type IV–VI) patterns have higher incidences of ligamentous injuries.

8.2 Meniscal injury

The incidence of meniscal injury associated with tibial plateau fractures based on preoperative MRI has been reported from 49 to 91% [47, 65–68]. Degree of lateral articular depression and condylar widening has been shown to directly correlate with frequency of soft tissue injuries in many studies [69–71]. Gardner et al. [72] in their MRI study on lateral split depression fractures found that articular depression >6 mm and condylar widening >5 mm was associated with a lateral meniscal injury 83% of the time. Stahl et al. [73] in their 661 patient intraoperative visualization study found that the most common Schatzker pattern associated with a lateral meniscus tear was the split depression fracture (45%) and the most common associated meniscal tear for this fracture pattern is peripheral rim avulsions (83%). 86% of Schatzker IV fractures had an associated medial meniscus tear [65].

8.3 Soft tissue diagnosis and treatment

Diagnosis of soft tissue injury based on physical exam findings is difficult due to the pain, swelling, and instability that is frequently present with these fractures. Recent studies have utilized preoperative MRI or operative arthroscopy to evaluate the extent of soft tissue damage. Treatment and pre-operative imaging protocols of ligamentous and meniscal pathology are controversial. Some authors advocate for MRI screening and surgical repair [47, 74, 75] whereas others have shown good results with no surgical intervention and advocate against MRI screening [67, 76–78]. Others argue against the use of pre-operative MRI because it overstates the true incidence of meniscal tears that require operative management, and instead they recommend direct visualization for lateral split depression fractures because the incidence of meniscal injury is sufficiently high enough to warrant this [73]. The clinical impact of identification of ligament and meniscal injuries is not clear from the current studies in the literature. Determining the functional impact would require a study that randomizes ligament treatment into surgical and nonsurgical groups. The literature does provide us with a clearer indication for nonoperative management on specific ligamentous injuries like MCL tears which can heal with nonoperative care with excellent functional outcomes. It remains controversial whether ACL or PCL surgical reattachment is indicated in the setting of tibial plateau fractures.

9. Nonsurgical treatment

Nonsurgical management is an option for certain fractures and specific clinical circumstances. Immediate passive range of motion with non-weight bearing for anywhere from 6 to 12 weeks in hinged bracing is currently preferred because it allows for mobility while maintaining coronal support. Indications for nonsurgical treatment include undisplaced or minimally displaced fractures, less than 5° of varus/valgus instability, delayed presentation, significant medical comorbidities precluding patients from operation, nonambulatory patients, and elderly patients with low functional status where deformities would be tolerated. Key to selecting patients for nonsurgical management is the ability to predict the post-treatment risk for deformity, malalignment, and instability. Angular malalignment is not well tolerated by patients and will cause cosmetic issues, articular cartilage overload, and increased likelihood of knee instability which can cause patients to be unbalanced and have an increased risk for falls. Risk for instability can be further assessed with a knowledge of the patient's demographics, activity level, comorbidities, and limb alignment. Imaging assessments that are helpful in assessing risk for instability include bone quality, fracture type, condylar width, degree of articular depression, and extent of fracture comminution.

Looking at the fracture pattern can further help your decision making. Larger lateral split depression fractures and all medial plateau fractures have a much higher propensity to collapse into valgus and varus deformity respectively whereas smaller fragment Schatzker II fractures can be amenable to nonsurgical management. Nearly all unicondylar medial tibial plateau fractures with displacement and displaced bicondylar fractures should be operated on [79].

Surgical treatment is commonly utilized in order to assure accurate limb alignment, gain early mobility, and achieve a better reduction. However, it behooves the clinician to remember that nonsurgical treatments can achieve excellent outcomes for patients unable or unwilling to undergo surgery despite articular incongruities and displacements [80].

10. Surgical treatment

Until the 1950s tibial plateau fractures were mostly treated nonoperatively with cast immobilization, however, operative treatment is currently the standard of care in the majority of tibial plateau fractures overall. The goals of surgical treatment of a tibial plateau fracture are to restore articular congruity, axial alignment, joint stability, and knee functionality. Fixation must be able to maintain stability postoperatively while allowing for early motion and minimizing complications.

10.1 Surgical indications

Operative management is indicated for tibial plateau fractures where near-anatomic alignment cannot predictably be achieved based on fracture pattern, physical exam findings, and radiographic measurements. In young active patients without comorbidities, fracture patterns that necessitate operative management include bicondylar plateau fractures and shaft dissociation patterns. Also, the majority of medial and lateral plateau fractures require surgical management unless they are minimally displaced and normal tibial/knee alignment can be achieved without fixation.

Another proposed indication for surgery is based on the amount of articular depression. This indication is more heavily debated and different cutoffs are found throughout the literature. Cutoffs for articular depression that result in poor outcomes if not operatively managed range from >2.5 to >10 mm [37, 38, 79, 81–85]. Unfortunately, the accuracy and reliability of measuring degree of articular depression is questionable. Martin et al. found that independent observers make articular depression measurements that differ by 12 mm or more 10% of the time [86]. Having a greater degree of articular depression than a predetermined cutoff should not be the sole basis for proceeding or not proceeding with surgery.

Poor functional outcomes and a high incidence of meniscal pathology have led many authors to suggest a condylar width increase of >5 mm and varus/valgus instability >5° as an indication for surgery [38, 72, 79]. However, Wang et al. [87] were unable to predict soft tissue injury based on tibial plateau widening. Johannsen et al. [14] suggest that discrepancies in the literature on condylar widening can be reconciled by instead using a ratio of the articular widths of the femur and tibia in order to minimize problems in measurement with magnification and calibration.

In the elderly, inactive or less active, or patients with comorbidities that place them at higher surgical risk, the decision whether to proceed with operative management needs to be more carefully assessed. A risk benefit analysis for each individual patient needs to be weighed in order to decide appropriate management. Elderly and the less active will be less affected by minor deformity if their functional demands are less.

10.2 Temporary external fixation

External fixation use has continued to evolve in the temporary and definitive management of these injuries. External fixation is commonly used as a temporary treatment by spanning the knee. This technique realigns and restores length allowing for soft tissue recovery prior to definitive treatment with internal fixation. Egol et al. [88] demonstrated the effectiveness of this technique with relatively low rates of complications in patients with high-energy tibial plateau fractures. With minimal soft tissue complications, the group recommended staged fixation for all high-energy fractures of the proximal tibia. Temporary external fixation not only provides skeletal stabilization to maintain length, alignment, and rotation, but also allows for easy access for wound and blister management. Studies have been performed, however, that show immediate fixation of most high energy tibial plateau fractures is safe and effective [89–91].

10.2.1 Definitive external fixation

Definitive external fixation typically uses a fine wire external fixator to compress against the fracture segments in conjunction with limited-access internal fixation which allows for minimal soft tissue disruption and permits early range of motion compared to ORIF with similar stabilization. Indications for definitive external fixation include severe open fractures and highly comminuted fractures where internal fixation is not possible. External fixation can also be used in conjunction with minimal internal fixation such as lag screws providing compression to the articular fragments. Multiple studies report equivocal rates of infections and complications when comparing ORIF and external fixation [76, 92, 93]. On the contrary, Krupp et al. [94] conducted a study comparing external fixation and open reduction of bicondylar tibial plateau fractures and they report significantly higher rates of malunion (7% vs. 40%), infections (7% vs. 13%), knee stiffness (4% vs. 13%) and overall complications (27% vs. 48%) of external fixation compared to ORIF. Shao et al. [56] also report significantly higher surgical site infection rates with external fixation.

10.2.2 Pin site placement for external fixation

Pin site placement and its importance varies between surgeons and in the literature. Classically, it is recommended that pins should be placed outside the zone of future plate placement and at least 14 mm distal to the joint line to avoid penetration into the joint [95]. However, there is new conflicting data on whether this has any effect at all on infection rate. Labile et al. [96] found no increased infection rate whereas Shah et al. [97] found the opposite. However, until we have a larger study to give us a definitive answer the recommendation is to place pin sites outside of the zone of injury in the case of temporary external fixation, and outside of the knee capsular reflection when placing wires for definitive treatment. With that being said, these recommendations should not outweigh the goal of achieving restoration of length, alignment, and stability of the fracture regardless of plans for future surgery.

10.3 Open reduction internal fixation (ORIF)

Open Reduction internal fixation (ORIF) is the most commonly used operative treatment for tibial plateau fractures. Multiple surgical approaches have been described in the surgical treatment of tibial plateau fractures. Anterolateral and posteromedial are the two surgical approaches that are most commonly used to reduce and internally fix tibial plateau fractures. They are used either together or in isolation depending on the fracture pattern. Dual incision approach is as effective in obtaining reduction and much safer than extensile approaches with no significant increase in infection rates seen [54, 98]. There are also multiple other posterior approaches described in the literature that have become popular. The fracture pattern is the main determinant of the approach and fixation technique. Direct anterior approaches can be helpful in conjunction with parapatellar arthrotomy in order to gain direct visualization and access to a greater area of the articular surface, especially centrally. It is important to note that when a direct anterior approach is used, soft tissue dissection should only proceed in one direction, medial or lateral from the incision. Anterior midline approaches with large dissection medial and lateral on the plateau are not recommended due to the devascularization caused to the plateau itself.

Plates and screws are the most common implants used in the fixation of tibial plateau fractures. Manufacturers have available pre-contoured periarticular plates as well as locking plates that are designed to fit against the proximal tibial surface. The plates can serve different functions depending on the anatomic placement and fracture pattern. Anterolateral plate placement in split depression fractures allows the plate to act as a buttress of the lateral tibial condyle supporting the weakened lateral cortex. On the other hand posteromedial plate placement functions as an antiglide device that resists shearing forces. Precontoured medial plates are also available from some manufacturers. Recently, plates have become thinner and both lateral and medial plates are most commonly 3.5 mm instead of the previous 4.5 mm. This allows the plates to fit closer to the bone and the corresponding 3.5 mm screws can be placed closer to the articular surface to better support reduced fragments. The plates also allow for subchondral screws to be placed parallel to the articular surface through the head of the plate, termed "rafting" (**Figure 8**), to significantly minimize postoperative articular depression [99]. Medially, plate position is more important than screw placement. The plate position must be closely intimate to the apex of the fracture and a screw near the apex of the fracture will help to ensure close apposition of the plate in this critical area.

Lateral plates alone can occasionally be used for bicondylar and Schatzker type VI fractures (**Figure 9**). These plates must resist axial, rotational, and bending force. The addition of locking screws to the plate has been a major advance in moving away from dual plating in some instances. Bending forces tend to create a varus deformity, however, and this must be considered if planning on using a single lateral plate in a bicondylar fracture pattern. Decreasing this varus collapse with fixed angle devices has decreased the need for dual plating in some instances, but this alone may be insufficient for providing adequate support for an unstable medial column. Although locking technology is available for most tibial plateau specific implants, its use in unicondylar fractures for buttress or antiglide plates is of unknown significance.

A special consideration must be taken for posterior plateau fragments which may not be adequately buttressed by medial or lateral plating. Involvement of the posterior segment has been shown to be more prevalent than previously recognized and failure to identify and manage it has been associated with misalignment and functional instability [22, 32, 100]. This could also be one of the reasons for failure in some fractures that still collapse secondarily after fixation [98, 101]. The use of the three column concept [19–21] may help in adequately addressing these fractures.

10.4 Void filling

Articular depression fractures (i.e., Schatzker II and III) result in a loss of cancellous bone volume due to the compression of cancellous trabeculae (**Figure 10A**). As a result of this, reduction of depressed tibial plateau articular fragments leads to an area void of bone underneath the reduced fragment (**Figure 10B** and **C**).These fragments in turn need to be adequately supported in order to reduce the risk of redisplacement. Metaphyseal void filling in these fracture patterns can be done to reduce this risk and to increase stability (**Figure 10D**).

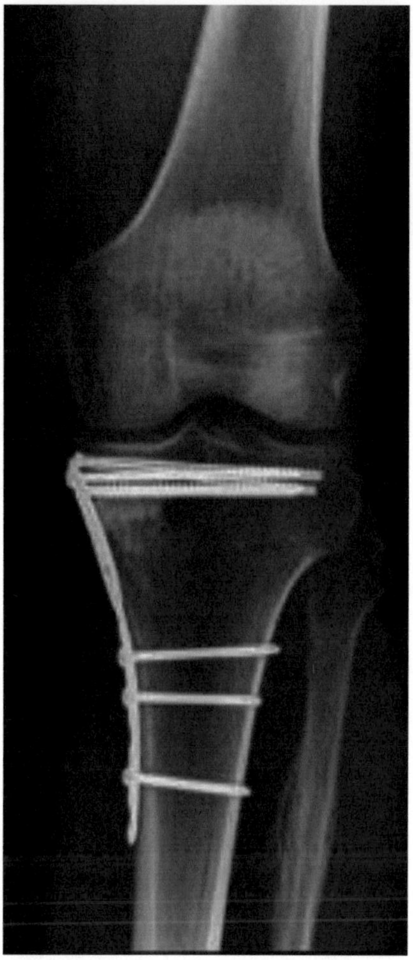

Figure 8.
AP radiograph of a medial tibial plateau fracture treated by ORIF with a medial buttress plate (Radiograph courtesy of John Riehl MD).

A wide range of options for materials to fill these voids are available. Autograft bone can be used, but supply is limited, extra surgical time is required, and there is associated morbidity at donor sites. Complications range from temporary pain or numbness, superficial infections, seromas, and minor hematomas to chronic pain, herniation of abdominal contents through donor sites at the pelvis, vascular injuries, deep infections, neurologic injuries, deep hematomas and iliac wing fractures.

Allografts have the advantage of no donor site morbidity and increased quantity available from bone banks. Osteogenesis, osteoinduction and osteoconduction are benefits and properties of autografts whereas only osteoconduction and poorer osteoinduction are provided by most allografts. As a result, the healing of allografts is often slower than the healing that occurs with autograft. The possibility of donor disease transmission exists but this risk is significantly reduced with donor screening and tissue testing. Segur et al. [102] found no complication secondary to the allograft transplantation in their short term follow up study (non-union, infection, fracture, resorption and transmission of disease).

Several commercially available graft substitutes are now used in the treatment of tibial plateau fractures. Most recently, phase-changing cements have shown promising results with better mechanical properties to autologous and allogenic bone grafts. Calcium phosphate cement was significantly stiffer and displayed significantly less

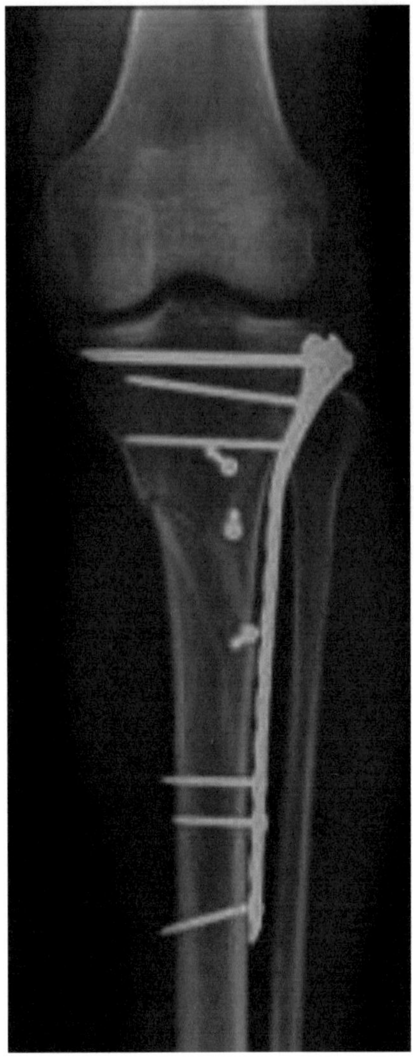

Figure 9.
AP radiograph of a Schatzker VI tibial plateau fracture treated by ORIF with a lateral plate and three independent lag screws (Radiograph courtesy of John Riehl MD).

displacement at 1000 N when compared to cancellous bone in a split depression fracture cadaver model study [103]. Lobenhoffer et al. [104] noted improved radiographic outcomes and earlier weight bearing due to its high mechanical strength. Russell et al. [105] noted a significantly higher rate of articular subsidence during the 3- to 12-month follow-up period in the autogenous bone graft group compared with the calcium phosphate group in their 119-patient study that included all six Schatzker patterns. Welch et al. [106] found similar results in their study comparing autologous bone graft with calcium phosphate in lateral articular depression fractures in goats. They found the autograft did not maintain anatomic reductions and calcium phosphate had significantly reduced fracture subsidence compared to the autograft at all time points. Recently, the use of calcium phosphate has also shown improved results in complex tibial plateau fractures (**Figure 11**) with significantly lower rates of articular step-off [107].

Another option that has been recently studied is beta-tricalciumphosphate which is a synthetic bone substitute that is biocompatible, biomechanically stable, and osteoconductive. Rolvien et al. [33] studied the long term results in tibial plateau depression fractures that used beta-tricalciumphosphate. They found no

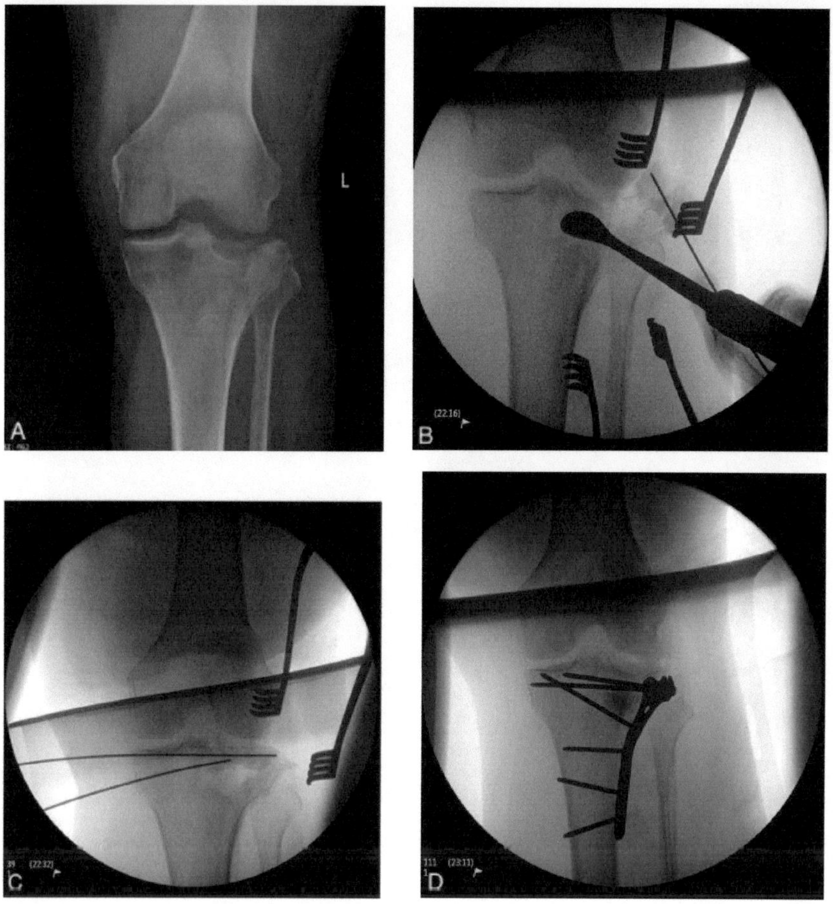

Figure 10.
Preoperative AP (A) X-ray of a Schatzker II split depression fracture. Intraoperative fluoroscopy shows elevation of the articular segment with a Cobb elevator (B), provisionally stabilized with K-wires creating a metaphyseal void (C). Final intraoperative imaging shows the reduced fracture with a lateral plate and calcium phosphate void filling cement (D) (Radiographs courtesy of John Riehl MD).

non-union or loss of reduction at a mean of 36 months of follow up. About 83% of patients achieved excellent reduction with <2 mm residual incongruity and 82% of patients achieved excellent functional outcomes. Histologic analysis of 7 of the patients demonstrated incorporation of bone around the graft but complete resorption was not observed. They concluded that beta-tricalciumphosphate represents an effective and safe treatment for these fractures, but its biological degradation and replacement is less pronounced in humans compared with previous animal studies.

Calcium sulfate has also been used as a void filler. Yu et al. [108] followed 28 patients for a mean of 14.6 months after using calcium sulfate as a void filler and found that 67% of the graft material was incorporated at 8 weeks and full incorporation was seen at 12 weeks. Fractures healed in all patients, and no nonunion or infection occurred. Wound exudations were observed in two cases, and the wound healed in 2–3 weeks with wound dressing. However, Goff et al. [109] showed possible reason for caution with the use of calcium sulfate in their more recent meta-analysis including 672 patients, comparing multiple void filling substitutes. They reported secondary collapse of the knee joint surface ≥2 mm in 8.6% in the biological substitutes (allograft, demineralized bone matrix, and xenograft), 5.4% in the hydroxyapatite, 3.7% in the calcium phosphate cement, and 11.1% in the calcium sulfate cases. It should be noted that the sample size of the calcium sulfate cases in this study was <40.

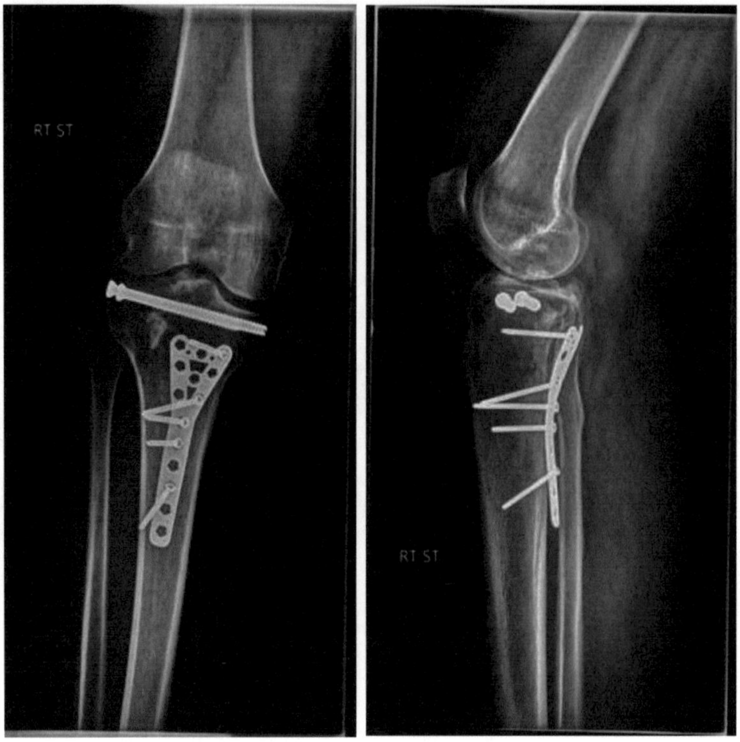

Figure 11.
AP and lateral X-ray showing reduction and fixation of a bicondylar tibial plateau fracture with posteromedial buttress plating, lateral lag screws, and quickset calcium phosphate (Radiographs courtesy of John Riehl MD).

Biphasic bone grafts that include calcium sulfate may give better results than calcium sulfate alone. A 2020 prospective, randomized control, multicenter study was conducted by Hofmann et al. [110] comparing autologous iliac bone graft to biphasic hydroxyapatite and calcium sulfate cement (60% calcium sulfate and 40% hydroxyapatite) in tibial plateau fractures. They concluded that the bioresorbable cement used was noninferior in both patient reported and radiographic outcomes to autologous bone graft in tibial plateau fractures.

10.5 Minimally invasive plate osteosynthesis (MIPO)

MIPO is a plating technique that enables indirect fracture reduction and percutaneous submuscular implant placement which improves healing rate due to its minimal disruption of soft tissues, including the periosteum and its vascularity [111–113]. Farouk et al. performed a cadaver study comparing post-procedure bone blood supplies in conventional plate osteosynthesis versus MIPO. Perforating and nutrient arteries remained intact and better periosteal and medullary perfusion was observed in the MIPO group compared to conventional plating [113]. ORIF allows for direct visualization, reduction, and fixation, but it is at the cost of substantial soft tissue dissection, increased risk of wound breakdown, stiffness, and deep infections [114]. Surgical techniques can provide benefits of both ORIF and MIPO techniques with the utilization of a small incision near the joint line with direct visualization and fixation of the joint while simultaneously performing percutaneous minimally invasive techniques in placement and securing the shaft portion of a plate. While some surgeons prefer to place percutaneous screws with use of fluoroscopy and feel, percutaneous guides can assist in efficient and accurate placement of shaft screws in these plates.

10.6 Intramedullary nailing

Intramedullary nailing (IMN) has many advantages for fracture fixation. These include minimally invasive exposure, biologically friendly implant insertion, longer implants to span more complex fractures, and load sharing fixation that allows for earlier weight bearing. With previous implants, concern for malreduction with intra-articular fractures was due to the nails inherent design flaws that failed to align properly with metaphyseal and epiphyseal segments. Recent advances in the implants have placed multiplanar interlocking screws clustered near the ends of nails to facilitate greater purchase in proximal segments and the ability to lock the interlocking screws to the nail creating a fixed angle construct which theoretically improves stability [115]. With these new improvements intramedullary nailing can be safely used to

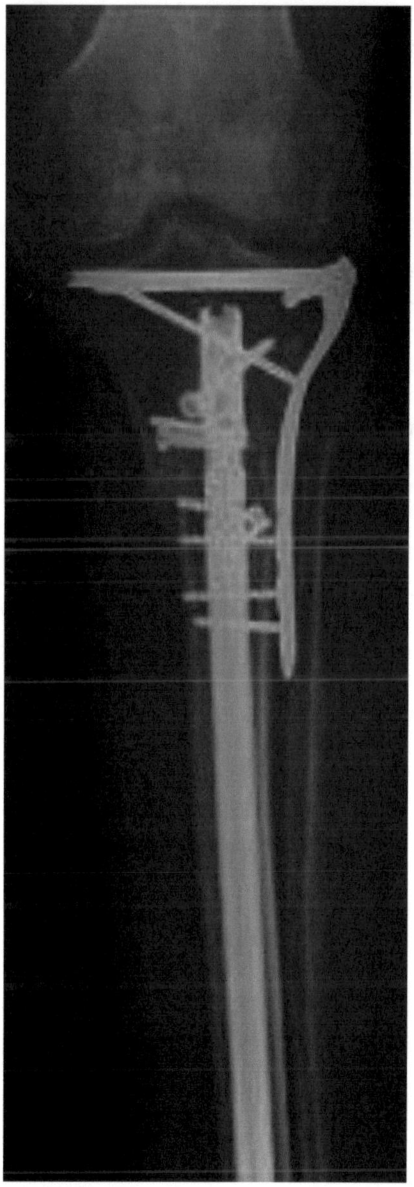

Figure 12.
Tibial plateau fracture with diaphyseal extension treated with a combination of lateral buttress plating and a tibial nail (Radiograph courtesy of John Riehl MD).

stabilize proximal intra-articular tibial fractures in which a stable articular block can be created. Often, this is performed by placement of independent lag screws proximally and outside of the intended path for the nail, or with buttress plating used with techniques compatible with nailing (**Figure 12**). Intramedullary nailing can especially be considered in tibial fracture patterns with diaphyseal extension, segmental injuries, or patients with increased risk for wound complications [115, 116]. Patients at increased risk for wound complications include patients with morbid obesity, diabetes, peripheral vascular disease, thin skin and compromised soft tissues. Prior to nailing, fractures should be converted from C-type articular fractures to A-type fractures by obtaining anatomic reduction and stable fixation of the articular surface. Contraindications to nailing may include tibial tubercle involvement in the fracture pattern and inability to reconstruct the articular surface outside of the planned nail trajectory. Fractures with tibial tuberosity fragments are poor candidates because the nail can cause a substantial anteriorly directed deforming force [115].

Intramedullary nailing reliably leads to excellent outcomes when performed for appropriate indications. In a multi-center case series Yoon et al. [117] found excellent outcomes with the use of adjunct plate fixation prior to IMN for complex tibial plateau fractures with 93% (25/27) achieving bony union and no late fracture displacement reported. Jia et al. [118] had similar excellent outcomes in their cohort with no incidences of malunion, nonunion, or infection. Meena et al. [119] randomized proximal metaphyseal tibia fractures to lateral percutaneous locked plating versus IMN. The IMN group had significantly shorter average hospital stay, time to fracture union, and time to full weight bearing. No significant difference was found for infection rate, range of motion of the knee or degrees of malunion and nonunion.

11. Postoperative treatment

11.1 Bracing

Bracing postoperatively is common practice with rigid braces holding the knee in extension, or more commonly hinged braces used for 3–6 weeks [120]. However, a recent prospective trial conducted by Chauhan et al. [121] found no significant difference between 6 weeks of bracing and no bracing at all after ORIF of tibial plateau fractures for union rates, postoperative range of motion, and Medical Outcomes Study 36-Item Short Form scores.

11.2 Weight bearing

Full weight-bearing is commonly delayed for 9–12 weeks with 4–6 weeks of non-weight bearing followed by 4–6 weeks of partial weight-bearing [120]. Two recent retrospective articles with sample sizes of 17 and 90 have challenged this notion with excellent results with immediate full weight bearing as tolerated [122, 123]. Basic science evidence supports a period of protected weight bearing followed by progressive loading due to evidence that gentle compressive loading may positively impact articular cartilage healing by improving chondrocyte survival, but excessive shearing may be detrimental [124]. More robust research is likely needed before major changes in weight-bearing protocols are implemented.

11.3 Surgical site infection

A 2019 meta-analysis including 7925 patients found the incidence of superficial and deep surgical site infections after tibial plateau fracture repairs to be 4.2% and 5.9%, respectively [55]. Risk factors that have been found to be associated with surgical site infections include open fractures [54–56, 125], compartment syndrome [27, 54–56], smoking [55, 56, 125], alcohol intake [126], definitive external fixation [56, 94] and intraoperative duration approaching 3 h [54, 56, 125]. A recent article found a strong correlation between a significantly higher peak of C-reactive protein (CRP) >100 μg/mL on postoperative day 3 and the development of surgical site infections in tibial plateau patients [127]. This finding might be an indication for more close surveillance in these patients regardless of CRP normalization over the following days, especially if the patient is at increased risk for noncompliance (e.g., Dementia).

11.4 Posttraumatic arthritis

The incidence of knee osteoarthritis following tibial plateau fractures reported in the literature has a wide range from 13 to 83% [6, 37, 38, 83, 84, 128–134]. Associated risk factors of early onset knee arthritis include degree of comminution, bicondylar fractures, meniscectomy, axial malalignment, joint instability, and older age [83, 85, 135, 136]. Wasserstein et al. [136], reporting on 8426 tibial plateau fractures, found that 7.3% of patients underwent total knee arthroplasty (TKA) 10 years after surgical management of tibial plateau fractures compared to only 1.8% in their control group. However, only adult patients treated by open reduction internal fixation (ORIF) were included and young patients and patients managed by conservative means or external fixation were excluded. Elsoe et al. [137] studied 7950 tibial plateau fracture patients in a matched cohort study and found the rate of TKA after tibial plateau fracture was 5.7% compared to 2% in their reference group.

12. Conclusion

Tibial plateau fractures comprise a wide range of fracture patterns, injury severity, and can exist with the presence or absence of significant associated injuries. History, physical exam, and imaging modalities can help to determine management of this complex category of injuries. Surgical and nonsurgical treatments can be employed to achieve healing and satisfactory long term results. Emerging technologies and implants continue to provide the promise of improved patient outcomes.

Author details

Christian M. Schmidt II [1], Jan P. Szatkowski[1] and John T. Riehl[2*]

1 Indiana University School of Medicine, Indianapolis, United States of America

2 Coastal Orthopaedic Trauma, FL, United States of America

*Address all correspondence to: jtriehl@hotmail.com

References

[1] Court-Brown CM, Caesar B. Epidemiology of adult fractures: A review. Injury. 2006;**37**(8):691-697

[2] Moore TM, Patzakis MJ, Harvey JP. Tibial plateau fractures: Definition, demographics, treatment rationale, and long-term results of closed traction management or operative reduction. Journal of Orthopaedic Trauma. 1987;**1**(2):97-119

[3] Albuquerque RP, el Hara R, Prado J, Schiavo L, Giordano V. do Amaral NP. Epidemiological study on tibial plateau fractures at a level i trauma center. Acta Ortopédica Brasileira. 2013;**21**(2):109-115

[4] Yuwen P, Lv H, Chen W, Wang Y, Yu Y, Hao J, et al. Age-, gender- and Arbeitsgemeinschaft fur Osteosynthesefragen type-specific clinical characters of adult tibial plateau fractures in eighty three hospitals in China. International Orthopaedics. 2018;**42**(3):667-672

[5] Elsoe R, Larsen P, Nielsen NPH, Swenne J, Rasmussen S, Ostgaard SE. Population-based epidemiology of tibial plateau fractures. Orthopedics. 2015;**38**(9):e780-e786

[6] Ebraheim NA, Sabry FF, Haman SP. Open reduction and internal fixation of 117 tibial plateau fractures. Orthopedics. 2004;**27**(12):1281-1287

[7] Blokker CP, Rorabeck CH, Bourne RB. Tibial plateau fractures. An analysis of the results of treatment in 60 patients. Clinical Orthopaedics and Related Research. 1984;**182**:193-199

[8] Kugelman DN, Qatu AM, Strauss EJ, Konda SR, Egol KA. Knee stiffness after Tibial plateau fractures: Predictors and outcomes (OTA-41). Journal of Orthopaedic Trauma. 2018;**32**(11):e421-e4e7

[9] He QF, Sun H, Shu LY, Zhan Y, He CY, Zhu Y, et al. Tibial plateau fractures in elderly people: An institutional retrospective study. Journal of Orthopaedic Surgery and Research. 2018;**13**(1):276

[10] Anderson DD, Mosqueda T, Thomas T, Hermanson EL, Brown TD, Marsh JL. Quantifying tibial plafond fracture severity: Absorbed energy and fragment displacement agree with clinical rank ordering. Journal of Orthopaedic Research. 2008;**26**(8):1046-1052

[11] Kugelman D, Qatu A, Haglin J, Leucht P, Konda S, Egol K. Complications and unplanned outcomes following operative treatment of tibial plateau fractures. Injury [Internet]. 2017;**48**(10):2221-2229

[12] Kennedy JC, Bailey WH. Experimental tibial-plateau fractures. Studies of the mechanism and a classification. The Journal of Bone and Joint Surgery. American Volume. 1968;**50A**(8):1522-1534

[13] Thamyongkit S, Fayad LM, Jones LC, Hasenboehler EA, Sirisreetreerux N, Shafiq B. The distal femur is a reliable guide for tibial plateau fracture reduction: A study of measurements on 3D CT scans in 84 healthy knees. Journal of Orthopaedic Surgery and Research. 2018;**13**(1):224

[14] Johannsen AM, Cook AM, Gardner MJ, Bishop JA. Defining the width of the normal tibial plateau relative to the distal femur: Critical normative data for identifying pathologic widening in tibial plateau fractures. Clinical Anatomy. 2018;**31**(5):688-692

[15] Hashemi J, Chandrashekar N, Gill B, Beynnon BD, Slauterbeck JR, Schutt RC, et al. The geometry of the tibial plateau

and its influence on the biomechanics of the tibiofemoral joint. The Journal of Bone and Joint Surgery - Series A. 2008;**90**(12):2724-2734

[16] Moore TM, Harvey JP Jr. Roentgenographic measurement of tibial-plateau depression due to fracture. The Journal of Bone and Joint Surgery. American Volume. 1974;**56**(1):155-160

[17] Weinberg DS, Williamson DF, Gebhart JJ, Knapik DM, Voos JE. Differences in medial and lateral posterior tibial slope: An osteological review of 1090 tibiae comparing age, sex, and race. The American Journal of Sports Medicine. 2017;**45**(1):106-113

[18] Schatzker J, McBroom R, Bruce D. The tibial plateau fracture. The Toronto experience 1968-1975. Clinical Orthopaedics and Related Research. 1979;(138):94-104

[19] Luo CF, Sun H, Zhang B, Zeng BF. Three-column fixation for complex tibial plateau fractures. Journal of Orthopaedic Trauma. 2010;**24**(11):683-692

[20] Zhu Y, Yang G, Luo CF, Smith WR, Hu CF, Gao H, et al. Computed tomography-based three-column classification in tibial plateau fractures: Introduction of its utility and assessment of its reproducibility. Journal of Trauma and Acute Care Surgery. 2012;**73**(3):731-737

[21] Wang Y, Luo C, Zhu Y, Zhai Q, Zhan Y, Qiu W, et al. Updated three-column concept in surgical treatment for tibial plateau fractures—A prospective cohort study of 287 patients. Injury. 2016;**47**(7):1488-1496

[22] Yang G, Zhai Q, Zhu Y, Sun H, Putnis S, Luo C. The incidence of posterior tibial plateau fracture: An investigation of 525 fractures by using a CT-based classification system. Archives of Orthopaedic and Trauma Surgery. 2013;**133**(7):929-934

[23] Hua K, Jiang X, Zha Y, Chen C, Zhang B, Mao Y. Retrospective analysis of 514 cases of tibial plateau fractures based on morphology and injury mechanism. Journal of Orthopaedic Surgery and Research. 2019;**14**(1):267

[24] Wahlquist M, Iaguilli N, Ebraheim N, Levine J. Medial tibial plateau fractures: A new classification system. The Journal of Trauma. 2007;**63**(6):1418-1421

[25] Stark E, Stucken C, Trainer G, Tornetta P 3rd. Compartment syndrome in Schatzker type VI plateau fractures and medial condylar fracture-dislocations treated with temporary external fixation. Journal of Orthopaedic Trauma. 2009;**23**(7):502-506

[26] Allmon C, Greenwell P, Paryavi E, Dubina A, O'Toole RV. Radiographic predictors of compartment syndrome occurring after tibial fracture. Journal of Orthopaedic Trauma. 2016;**30**(7):387-391

[27] Blair JA, Stoops TK, Doarn MC, Kemper D, Erdogan M, Griffing R, et al. Infection and nonunion after fasciotomy for compartment syndrome associated with tibia fractures: A matched cohort comparison. Journal of Orthopaedic Trauma. 2016;**30**(7):392-396

[28] Marchand LS, Working ZM, Rane AA, Elliott IS, Gilbertson E, Rothberg DL, et al. Compartment syndrome in tibial plateau fractures: Do previously established predictors have external validity? Journal of Orthopaedic Trauma. 2019;**34**(5):238-243

[29] Gamulin A, Lubbeke A, Belinga P, Hoffmeyer P, Perneger TV, Zingg M, et al. Clinical and radiographic predictors of acute compartment syndrome in the treatment of tibial

plateau fractures: A retrospective cohort study. BMC Musculoskeletal Disorders. 2017;**18**(1):307

[30] Moore TM. Fracture–dislocation of the knee. Clinical Orthopaedics and Related Research. 1981;**156**:128-140

[31] Fracture and Dislocation Compendium. Orthopaedic Trauma Association Committee for coding and classification. Journal of Orthopaedic Trauma. 1996;**10**(Suppl 1:v–ix):1-154

[32] Jiwanlal A, Jeray KJ. Outcome of posterior tibial plateau fixation. The Journal of Knee Surgery. 2016;**29**(1):34-39

[33] Rolvien T, Barvencik F, Klatte TO, Busse B, Hahn M, Rueger JM, et al. Ss-TCP bone substitutes in tibial plateau depression fractures. The Knee. 2017;**24**(5):1138-1145

[34] Halvorson JJ, Anz A, Langfitt M, Deonanan JK, Scott A, Teasdall RD, et al. Vascular injury associated with extremity trauma: Initial diagnosis and management. The Journal of the American Academy of Orthopaedic Surgeons. 2011;**19**(8):495-504

[35] Green NE, Allen BL. Vascular injuries associated with dislocation of the knee. The Journal of Bone and Joint Surgery. American Volume. 1977;**59**(2):236-239

[36] Stayner LR, Coen MJ. Historic perspectives of treatment algorithms in knee dislocation. Clinics in Sports Medicine. 2000;**19**(3):399-413

[37] Rasmussen PS. Tibial condylar fractures. Impairment of knee joint stability as an indication for surgical treatment. The Journal of Bone and Joint Surgery. American Volume. 1973;**55**(7):1331-1350

[38] Lansinger O, Bergman B, Korner L, Andersson GB. Tibial condylar fractures. A twenty-year follow-up. The Journal of Bone and Joint Surgery. American Volume. 1986;**68**(1):13-19

[39] Prasad N, Murray JM, Kumar D, Davies SG. Insufficiency fracture of the tibial plateau: An often missed diagnosis. Acta Orthopaedica Belgica. 2006;**72**(5):587-591

[40] Chan PS, Klimkiewicz JJ, Luchetti WT, Esterhai JL, Kneeland JB, Dalinka MK, et al. Impact of CT scan on treatment plan and fracture classification of tibial plateau fractures. Journal of Orthopaedic Trauma. 1997;**11**(7):484-489

[41] Wicky S, Blaser PF, Blanc CH, Leyvraz PF, Schnyder P, Meuli RA. Comparison between standard radiography and spiral CT with 3D reconstruction in the evaluation, classification and management of tibial plateau fractures. European Radiology. 2000;**10**(8):1227-1232

[42] Macarini L, Murrone M, Marini S, Calbi R, Solarino M, Moretti B. Tibial plateau fractures: Evaluation with multidetector-CT. La Radiologia Medica. 2004;**108**(5-6):503-514

[43] Markhardt BK, Gross JM, Monu JU. Schatzker classification of tibial plateau fractures: Use of CT and MR imaging improves assessment. Radiographics. 2009;**29**(2):585-597

[44] Brunner A, Horisberger M, Ulmar B, Hoffmann A, Babst R. Classification systems for tibial plateau fractures; does computed tomography scanning improve their reliability? Injury. 2010;**41**(2):173-178

[45] Molenaars RJ, Mellema JJ, Doornberg JN, Kloen P. Tibial plateau fracture characteristics: Computed tomography mapping of lateral, medial, and bicondylar fractures. The Journal of Bone and Joint Surgery. American Volume. 2015;**97**(18):1512-1520

[46] Liow RY, Birdsall PD, Mucci B, Greiss ME. Spiral computed tomography with two- and three-dimensional reconstruction in the management of tibial plateau fractures. Orthopedics. 1999;**22**(10):929-932

[47] Stannard JP, Lopez R, Volgas D. Soft tissue injury of the knee after tibial plateau fractures. The Journal of Knee Surgery. 2010;**23**(4):187-192

[48] Mui LW, Engelsohn E, Umans H. Comparison of CT and MRI in patients with tibial plateau fracture: Can CT findings predict ligament tear or meniscal injury? Skeletal Radiology. 2007;**36**(2):145-151

[49] Vaillancourt C, Shrier I, Vandal A, Falk M, Rossignol M, Vernec A, et al. Acute compartment syndrome: How long before muscle necrosis occurs? CJEM. 2004;**6**(3):147-154

[50] Menetrey J, Peter R. Acute compartment syndrome in the post traumatic leg. Revue de Chirurgie Orthopédique et Réparatrice de l'Appareil Moteur. 1998;**84**(3):272-280

[51] Park S, Ahn J, Gee AO, Kuntz AF, Esterhai JL. Compartment syndrome in tibial fractures. Journal of Orthopaedic Trauma. 2009;**23**(7):514-518

[52] Ziran BH, Becher SJ. Radiographic predictors of compartment syndrome in tibial plateau fractures. Journal of Orthopaedic Trauma. 2013;**27**(11):612-615

[53] Andrews JR, Tedder JL, Godbout BP. Bicondylar tibial plateau fracture complicated by compartment syndrome. Orthopaedic Review. 1992;**21**(3):317-319

[54] Colman M, Wright A, Gruen G, Siska P, Pape HC, Tarkin I. Prolonged operative time increases infection rate in tibial plateau fractures. Injury. 2013;**44**(2):249-252

[55] Norris GR, Checketts JX, Scott JT, Vassar M, Norris BL, Giannoudis PV. Prevalence of deep surgical site infection after repair of periarticular knee fractures: A systematic review and meta-analysis. JAMA Network Open. 2019;**2**(8):e199951

[56] Shao J, Chang H, Zhu Y, Chen W, Zheng Z, Zhang H, et al. Incidence and risk factors for surgical site infection after open reduction and internal fixation of tibial plateau fracture: A systematic review and meta-analysis. International Journal of Surgery. 2017;**41**:176-182

[57] Ruffolo MR, Gettys FK, Montijo HE, Seymour RB, Karunakar MA. Complications of high-energy bicondylar tibial plateau fractures treated with dual plating through 2 incisions. Journal of Orthopaedic Trauma. 2015;**29**(2):85-90

[58] Ulmer T. The clinical diagnosis of compartment syndrome of the lower leg: Are clinical findings predictive of the disorder? Journal of Orthopaedic Trauma. 2002;**16**(8):572-577

[59] Schmidt AH. Acute compartment syndrome. Injury. 2017;**48**(Suppl 1): S22-SS5

[60] Prayson MJ, Chen JL, Hampers D, Vogt M, Fenwick J, Meredick R. Baseline compartment pressure measurements in isolated lower extremity fractures without clinical compartment syndrome. The Journal of Trauma. 2006;**60**(5):1037-1040

[61] McQueen MM, Duckworth AD, Aitken SA, Court-Brown CM. The estimated sensitivity and specificity of compartment pressure monitoring for acute compartment syndrome. The Journal of Bone and Joint Surgery. American Volume. 2013;**95**(8):673-677

[62] Kakar S, Firoozabadi R, McKean J, Tornetta P 3rd. Diastolic blood pressure in patients with tibia fractures under anaesthesia: Implications for the diagnosis of compartment syndrome. Journal of Orthopaedic Trauma. 2007;**21**(2):99-103

[63] Heckman MM, Whitesides TE Jr, Grewe SR, Rooks MD. Compartment pressure in association with closed tibial fractures. The relationship between tissue pressure, compartment, and the distance from the site of the fracture. The Journal of Bone and Joint Surgery. American Volume. 1994;**76**(9):1285-1292

[64] Nakhostine M, Styf JR, van Leuven S, Hargens AR, Gershuni DH. Intramuscular pressure varies with depth. The tibialis anterior muscle studied in 12 volunteers. Acta Orthopaedica Scandinavica. 1993;**64**(3):377-381

[65] Gardner MJ, Yacoubian S, Geller D, Suk M, Mintz D, Potter H, et al. The incidence of soft tissue injury in operative tibial plateau fractures: A magnetic resonance imaging analysis of 103 patients. Journal of Orthopaedic Trauma. 2005;**19**(2):79-84

[66] Shepherd L, Abdollahi K, Lee J, Vangsness CT Jr. The prevalence of soft tissue injuries in nonoperative tibial plateau fractures as determined by magnetic resonance imaging. Journal of Orthopaedic Trauma. 2002;**16**(9):628-631

[67] Warner SJ, Garner MR, Schottel PC, Fabricant PD, Thacher RR, Loftus ML, et al. The effect of soft tissue injuries on clinical outcomes after tibial plateau fracture fixation. Journal of Orthopaedic Trauma. 2018;**32**(3):141-147

[68] Colletti P, Greenberg H, Terk MR. MR findings in patients with acute tibial plateau fractures. Computerized Medical Imaging and Graphics. 1996;**20**(5):389-394

[69] Ringus VM, Lemley FR, Hubbard DF, Wearden S, Jones DL. Lateral tibial plateau fracture depression as a predictor of lateral meniscus pathology. Orthopedics. 2010;**33**(2):80-84

[70] Spiro AS, Regier M, Novo de Oliveira A, Vettorazzi E, Hoffmann M, Petersen JP, et al. The degree of articular depression as a predictor of soft-tissue injuries in tibial plateau fracture. Knee Surgery, Sports Traumatology, Arthroscopy. 2013;**21**(3):564-570

[71] Durakbasa MO, Kose O, Ermis MN, Demirtas A, Gunday S, Islam C. Measurement of lateral plateau depression and lateral plateau widening in a Schatzker type II fracture can predict a lateral meniscal injury. Knee Surgery, Sports Traumatology, Arthroscopy. 2013;**21**(9):2141-2146

[72] Gardner MJ, Yacoubian S, Geller D, Pode M, Mintz D, Helfet DL, et al. Prediction of soft-tissue injuries in Schatzker II tibial plateau fractures based on measurements of plain radiographs. The Journal of Trauma. 2006;**60**(2):319-323. discussion 24

[73] Stahl D, Serrano-Riera R, Collin K, Griffing R, Defenbaugh B, Sagi HC. Operatively treated meniscal tears associated with tibial plateau fractures: A report on 661 patients. Journal of Orthopaedic Trauma. 2015;**29**(7):322-324

[74] Bennett WF, Browner B. Tibial plateau fractures: A study of associated soft tissue injuries. Journal of Orthopaedic Trauma. 1994;**8**(3):183-188

[75] Lubowitz JH, Elson WS, Guttmann D. Part I: Arthroscopic management of tibial plateau fractures. Arthroscopy. 2004;**20**(10):1063-1070

[76] Canadian Orthopaedic Trauma Society. Open reduction and internal fixation compared with circular fixator application for bicondylar tibial plateau fractures. Results of a multicenter, prospective, randomized clinical trial. The Journal of Bone and Joint Surgery. American Volume. 2006;**88**(12):2613-2623

[77] Moore TM, Meyers MH, Harvey JP Jr. Collateral ligament laxity of the knee. Long-term comparison between plateau fractures and normal. The Journal of Bone and Joint Surgery. American Volume. 1976;**58**(5):594-598

[78] Elsoe R, Motahar I, Mahdi F, Larsen P. Presence of magnetic resonance imaging verified soft tissue injuries did not significantly affect the patient-reported outcome 12 months following a lateral tibial plateau fracture: A 12-month prospective cohort study of 56 patients. The Knee. 2020;**27**(2):420-427

[79] Honkonen SE. Indications for surgical treatment of tibial condyle fractures. Clinical Orthopaedics and Related Research. 1994;**302**:199-205

[80] Pean CA, Driesman A, Christiano A, Konda SR, Davidovitch R, Egol KA. Functional and clinical outcomes of nonsurgically managed tibial plateau fractures. The Journal of the American Academy of Orthopaedic Surgeons. 2017;**25**(5):375-380

[81] Waddell JP, Johnston DW, Neidre A. Fractures of the tibial plateau: A review of ninety-five patients and comparison of treatment methods. The Journal of Trauma. 1981;**21**(5):376-381

[82] Singleton N, Sahakian V, Muir D. Outcome after tibial plateau fracture: How important is restoration of articular congruity? Journal of Orthopaedic Trauma. 2017;**31**(3):158-163

[83] Parkkinen M, Madanat R, Mustonen A, Koskinen SK, Paavola M, Lindahl J. Factors predicting the development of early osteoarthritis following lateral tibial plateau fractures: Mid-term clinical and radiographic outcomes of 73 operatively treated patients. Scandinavian Journal of Surgery. 2014;**103**(4):256-262

[84] Jensen DB, Rude C, Duus B, Bjerg-Nielsen A. Tibial plateau fractures. A comparison of conservative and surgical treatment. Journal of Bone and Joint Surgery. British Volume (London). 1990;**72**(1):49-52

[85] Honkonen SE. Degenerative arthritis after tibial plateau fractures. Journal of Orthopaedic Trauma. 1995;**9**(4):273-277

[86] Martin J, Marsh JL, Nepola JV, Dirschl DR, Hurwitz S, DeCoster TA. Radiographic fracture assessments: Which ones can we reliably make? Journal of Orthopaedic Trauma. 2000;**14**(6):379-385

[87] Wang J, Wei J, Wang M. The distinct prediction standards for radiological assessments associated with soft tissue injuries in the acute tibial plateau fracture. European Journal of Orthopaedic Surgery and Traumatology. 2015;**25**(5):913-920

[88] Egol KA, Tejwani NC, Capla EL, Wolinsky PL, Koval KJ. Staged management of high-energy proximal tibia fractures (OTA types 41): The results of a prospective, standardized protocol. Journal of Orthopaedic Trauma. 2005;**19**(7):448-455; discussion 56

[89] Benirschke SK, Agnew SG, Mayo KA, Santoro VM, Henley MB. Immediate internal fixation of open, complex tibial plateau fractures: Treatment by a standard protocol. Journal of Orthopaedic Trauma. 1992;**6**(1):78-86

[90] Janes PC, Leonard J, Phillips JL, Bauer BJ, Salottolo K, Slone DS, et al.

Skiers and snowboarders have improved short-term outcomes with immediate fixation of tibial plateau fractures. Trauma Surgery & Acute Care Open. 2017;**2**(1):e000119

[91] Borade A, Kempegowda H, Richard R, Graham J, Suk M, Horwitz DS. Is "Early Total Care" a safe and effective alternative to "Staged Protocol" for the treatment of Schatzker IV-VI tibial plateau fractures in patients older than 50 years? Journal of Orthopaedic Trauma. 2017;**31**(12):e400-e4e6

[92] Metcalfe D, Hickson CJ, McKee L, Griffin XL. External versus internal fixation for bicondylar tibial plateau fractures: Systematic review and meta-analysis. Journal of Orthopaedics and Traumatology. 2015;**16**(4):275-285

[93] Mallik AR, Covall DJ, Whitelaw GP. Internal versus external fixation of bicondylar tibial plateau fractures. Orthopaedic Review. 1992;**21**(12):1433-1436

[94] Krupp RJ, Malkani AL, Roberts CS, Seligson D, Crawford CH 3rd, Smith L. Treatment of bicondylar tibia plateau fractures using locked plating versus external fixation. Orthopedics. 2009;**32**(8):559-566

[95] Reid JS, Van Slyke MA, Moulton MJ, Mann TA. Safe placement of proximal tibial transfixation wires with respect to intracapsular penetration. Journal of Orthopaedic Trauma. 2001;**15**(1):10-17

[96] Laible C, Earl-Royal E, Davidovitch R, Walsh M, Egol KA. Infection after spanning external fixation for high-energy tibial plateau fractures: Is pin site-plate overlap a problem? Journal of Orthopaedic Trauma. 2012;**26**(2):92-97

[97] Shah CM, Babb PE, McAndrew CM, Brimmo O, Badarudeen S, Tornetta P 3rd, et al. Definitive plates overlapping provisional external fixator pin sites: Is the infection risk increased? Journal of Orthopaedic Trauma. 2014;**28**(9):518-522

[98] Barei DP, Nork SE, Mills WJ, Henley MB, Benirschke SK. Complications associated with internal fixation of high-energy bicondylar tibial plateau fractures utilizing a two-incision technique. Journal of Orthopaedic Trauma. 2004;**18**(10):649-657

[99] Karunakar MA, Egol KA, Peindl R, Harrow ME, Bosse MJ, Kellam JF. Split depression tibial plateau fractures: A biomechanical study. Journal of Orthopaedic Trauma. 2002;**16**(3):172-177

[100] Quintens L, Van den Berg J, Reul M, Van Lieshout E, Nijs S, Verhofstad M, et al. Poor sporting abilities after tibial plateau fractures involving the posterior column: How can we do better? European Journal of Trauma and Emergency Surgery. 2019:1-9

[101] Gosling T, Schandelmaier P, Muller M, Hankemeier S, Wagner M, Krettek C. Single lateral locked screw plating of bicondylar tibial plateau fractures. Clinical Orthopaedics and Related Research. 2005;**439**:207-214

[102] Segur JM, Torner P, Garcia S, Combalia A, Suso S, Ramon R. Use of bone allograft in tibial plateau fractures. Archives of Orthopaedic and Trauma Surgery. 1998;**117**(6-7):357-359

[103] Trenholm A, Landry S, McLaughlin K, Deluzio KJ, Leighton J, Trask K, et al. Comparative fixation of tibial plateau fractures using alpha-BSM, a calcium phosphate cement, versus cancellous bone graft. Journal of Orthopaedic Trauma. 2005;**19**(10):698-702

[104] Lobenhoffer P, Gerich T, Witte F, Tscherne H. Use of an injectable calcium phosphate bone cement in the

treatment of tibial plateau fractures: A prospective study of twenty-six cases with twenty-month mean follow-up. Journal of Orthopaedic Trauma. 2002;**16**(3):143-149

[105] Russell TA, Leighton RK. Alpha BSMTPFSG. Comparison of autogenous bone graft and endothermic calcium phosphate cement for defect augmentation in tibial plateau fractures. A multicenter, prospective, randomized study. The Journal of Bone and Joint Surgery. American Volume. 2008;**90**(10):2057-2061

[106] Welch RD, Zhang H, Bronson DG. Experimental tibial plateau fractures augmented with calcium phosphate cement or autologous bone graft. The Journal of Bone and Joint Surgery. American Volume. 2003;**85**(2):222-231

[107] Ollivier M, Bulaid Y, Jacquet C, Pesenti S, Argenson JN, Parratte S. Fixation augmentation using calcium-phosphate bone substitute improves outcomes of complex tibial plateau fractures. A matched, cohort study. International Orthopaedics. 2018;**42**(12):2915-2923

[108] Yu B, Han K, Ma H, Zhang C, Su J, Zhao J, et al. Treatment of tibial plateau fractures with high strength injectable calcium sulphate. International Orthopaedics. 2009;**33**(4):1127-1133

[109] Goff T, Kanakaris NK, Giannoudis PV. Use of bone graft substitutes in the management of tibial plateau fractures. Injury. 2013;**44** (Suppl 1):S86-S94

[110] Hofmann A, Gorbulev S, Guehring T, Schulz AP, Schupfner R, Raschke M, et al. Autologous iliac bone graft compared with biphasic hydroxyapatite and calcium sulfate cement for the treatment of bone defects in tibial plateau fractures: A prospective, randomized, open-label, multicenter study. The Journal of Bone and Joint Surgery. American Volume. 2020;**102**(3):179-193

[111] Raza H, Hashmi P, Abbas K, Hafeez K. Minimally invasive plate osteosynthesis for tibial plateau fractures. Journal of Orthopaedic Surgery (Hong Kong). 2012;**20**(1):42-47

[112] Oh JK, Oh CW, Jeon IH, Kim SJ, Kyung HS, Park IH, et al. Percutaneous plate stabilization of proximal tibial fractures. The Journal of Trauma. 2005;**59**(2):431-437

[113] Farouk O, Krettek C, Miclau T, Schandelmaier P, Guy P, Tscherne H. Minimally invasive plate osteosynthesis: Does percutaneous plating disrupt femoral blood supply less than the traditional technique? Journal of Orthopaedic Trauma. 1999;**13**(6):401-406

[114] Lachiewicz PF, Funcik T. Factors influencing the results of open reduction and internal fixation of tibial plateau fractures. Clinical Orthopaedics and Related Research. 1990;**259**:210-215

[115] Virkus WW, Kempton LB, Sorkin AT, Gaski GE. Intramedullary nailing of periarticular fractures. The Journal of the American Academy of Orthopaedic Surgeons. 2018;**26**(18):629-639

[116] Natoli RM, Sardesai NR, Richard RD, Sorkin AT, Gaski GE, Virkus WW. Intramedullary nailing of lower-extremity periarticular fractures. JBJS Essential Surgical Techniques. 2019;**9**(4):e35.1-2

[117] Yoon RS, Bible J, Marcus MS, Donegan DJ, Bergmann KA, Siebler JC, et al. Outcomes following combined intramedullary nail and plate fixation for complex tibia fractures: A multi-centre study. Injury. 2015;**46**(6):1097-1101

[118] Jia P, Lu FC, Ullah K, Zhang M, Dong YS, Xiong C, et al. Angle stable interlocking intramedullary nails for tibial plateau fractures. Orthopaedic Surgery. 2018;**10**(2):115-120

[119] Meena RC, Meena UK, Gupta GL, Gahlot N, Gaba S. Intramedullary nailing versus proximal plating in the management of closed extra-articular proximal tibial fracture: A randomized controlled trial. Journal of Orthopaedics and Traumatology. 2015;**16**(3):203-208

[120] Arnold JB, Tu CG, Phan TM, Rickman M, Varghese VD, Thewlis D, et al. Characteristics of postoperative weight bearing and management protocols for tibial plateau fractures: Findings from a scoping review. Injury. 2017;**48**(12):2634-2642

[121] Chauhan A, Slipak A, Miller MC, Altman DT, Altman GT. No difference between bracing and no bracing after open reduction and internal fixation of tibial plateau fractures. The Journal of the American Academy of Orthopaedic Surgeons. 2018;**26**(6):e134-ee41

[122] Williamson M, Iliopoulos E, Jain A, Ebied W, Trompeter A. Immediate weight bearing after plate fixation of fractures of the tibial plateau. Injury. 2018;**49**(10):1886-1890

[123] Thewlis D, Fraysse F, Callary SA, Verghese VD, Jones CF, Findlay DM, et al. Postoperative weight bearing and patient reported outcomes at one year following tibial plateau fractures. Injury. 2017;**48**(7):1650-1656

[124] Irrgang JJ, Pezzullo D. Rehabilitation following surgical procedures to address articular cartilage lesions in the knee. The Journal of Orthopaedic and Sports Physical Therapy. 1998;**28**(4):232-240

[125] Li J, Zhu Y, Liu B, Dong T, Chen W, Zhang Y. Incidence and risk factors for surgical site infection following open reduction and internal fixation of adult tibial plateau fractures. International Orthopaedics. 2018;**42**(6):1397-1403

[126] Chan G, Iliopoulos E, Jain A, Turki M, Trompeter A. Infection after operative fixation of tibia plateau fractures. A risk factor analysis. Injury. 2019;**50**(11):2089-2092

[127] Ballhause TM, Krause M, Ross J, Rueger JM, Frosch KH, Klatte TO. Third day laboratory follow-up: Mandatory for surgical site infections of tibial plateau fractures. European Journal of Trauma and Emergency Surgery. 2019 [online ahead of print]

[128] Mehin R, O'Brien P, Broekhuyse H, Blachut P, Guy P. Endstage arthritis following tibia plateau fractures: Average 10-year follow-up. Canadian Journal of Surgery. 2012;**55**(2):87-94

[129] Manidakis N, Dosani A, Dimitriou R, Stengel D, Matthews S, Giannoudis P. Tibial plateau fractures: Functional outcome and incidence of osteoarthritis in 125 cases. International Orthopaedics. 2010;**34**(4):565-570

[130] Jansen H, Frey SP, Doht S, Fehske K, Meffert RH. Medium-term results after complex intra-articular fractures of the tibial plateau. Journal of Orthopaedic Science. 2013;**18**(4):569-577

[131] Scott CE, Davidson E, MacDonald DJ, White TO, Keating JF. Total knee arthroplasty following tibial plateau fracture: A matched cohort study. The Bone & Joint Journal. 2015;**97-B**(4):532-538

[132] DeCoster TA, Nepola JV, El-Khoury GY. Cast brace treatment of proximal tibia fractures. A ten-year follow-up study. Clinical Orthopaedics and Related Research. 1988;**231**:196-204

[133] Elsoe R, Larsen P, Shekhrajka N, Ferreira L, Ostgaard SE, Rasmussen S.

The outcome after lateral tibial plateau fracture treated with percutaneus screw fixation show a tendency towards worse functional outcome compared with a reference population. European Journal of Trauma and Emergency Surgery. 2016;**42**(2):177-184

[134] Elsoe R, Larsen P, Petruskevicius J, Kold S. Complex tibial fractures are associated with lower social classes and predict early exit from employment and worse patient-reported QOL: A prospective observational study of 46 complex tibial fractures treated with a ring fixator. Strategies in Trauma and Limb Reconstruction. 2018;**13**(1):25-33

[135] Rademakers MV, Kerkhoffs GM, Sierevelt IN, Raaymakers EL, Marti RK. Operative treatment of 109 tibial plateau fractures: Five- to 27-year follow-up results. Journal of Orthopaedic Trauma. 2007;**21**(1):5-10

[136] Wasserstein D, Henry P, Paterson JM, Kreder HJ, Jenkinson R. Risk of total knee arthroplasty after operatively treated tibial plateau fracture: A matched-population-based cohort study. The Journal of Bone and Joint Surgery. American Volume. 2014;**96**(2):144-150

[137] Elsoe R, Johansen MB, Larsen P. Tibial plateau fractures are associated with a long-lasting increased risk of total knee arthroplasty a matched cohort study of 7,950 tibial plateau fractures. Osteoarthritis and Cartilage. 2019;**27**(5):805-809

Chapter 2

Surgical Approaches and Leg Positions for Tibial Plateau Fractures

Katsimentzas Triantafyllos, Tryfon Ditsios and Kostantinos Ditsios

Abstract

Tibial plateau fractures are a common orthopedic injury. Epidemiological studies have shown that these injuries appear in younger or older patients with different mechanisms of injury. For better long-term results, it is crucial to achieve successful fracture reduction, thus avoiding the main complication, which is post-traumatic arthritis. Reduction can be achieved by choosing the proper surgical approach. Many approaches that address the fractures of the tibial plateau have been described in international literature. In the past, the direct anterior midline approach was used, which required a large detachment of the soft tissues. Nowadays, the percutaneous approach, the anterolateral approach, the medial approach, the posteromedial approach, the posterolateral approach, and the direct posterior approach are used by orthopedic surgeons to treat these kinds of fractures. In this chapter, we will describe the surgical approaches available for tibial plateau fractures and the possible positions of the affected leg.

Keywords: tibial plateau fractures, proximal tibia fractures, surgical approach, surgical incision, patient position, leg position

1. Introduction

Tibial plateau fractures constitute 1% of all bone fractures [1]. These intra-articular fractures are rare with an incidence of 10.3/100,000 per year [1]. They occur in young adults as a result of high energy trauma (motor accident, fall) or as low energy fractures in elderly patients with poor bone quality. This type of injury has a variety of fracture patterns. Compared to women, men younger than 50 years of age show a higher incidence for these fractures. Incidence increased markedly in women older than 50 years and decreased in men older than 50 years. For both sexes, the highest frequency was between ages 40 and 60 years [1].

Seventy percent of fractures are isolated to the lateral plateau, with 10–30% bicondylar and less than 10% isolated medial condyle fractures [2]. However, after multifragmentary articular surface destruction, they are often associated with a poor postoperative outcome [1]. With bicondylar fracture involvement, arthritis rates up to 44% have been described. Moreover, the medial plateau fractures with >3 mm displacement and anteromedial or posterolateral column fractures in young patients are associated with higher risk of ACL avulsion fracture [3].

Displaced fractures are treated with open reduction and internal fixation. The goals of treatment include restoration of extremity axial alignment, joint stability, and congruity, allowing early motion and prevention of osteoarthritis. Short-term results of surgical fixation of tibial plateau fractures are good; however, longer-term outcomes have demonstrated a significantly higher risk of end-stage arthritis and necessity for total knee arthroplasty [4].

Nontraumatic management of soft tissue with careful surgical incision is crucial in order to avoid further damage of the tissues around the fractured area. The choice of surgical approach is mainly based on the morphology of the fracture and the condition of the soft tissues, the general condition of the patient and the accompanying injuries. Computed tomography has greatly assisted in assessing the pattern of tibial plateau fractures.

It is important to achieve good reduction of the fracture for better long-term results with the proper surgical incision. The ideal surgery approach helps the orthopedic surgeon to evaluate the fracture and place the orthopedic fixation implants successfully.

2. Lateral approaches

2.1 Anterolateral approach

Lateral tibial plateau fractures are very common. Due to this reason, the anterolateral approach is the most frequently used surgical approach for tibial plateau fractures. This surgical incision can be used for simply split lateral tibial fractures with or without compression and also for comminuted bicondylar tibial fractures.

There are quite a few variations in skin incisions for the anterolateral approach. In this chapter, we will describe the two methods most commonly used. For the first one, the incision starts 2–3 cm proximal to the joint line and ends 3 cm inferior of the tibial tubercle, depending on the fracture pattern. This lazy "s" shaped incision begins directly lateral over the iliotibial band (IT), curves over Gerdy's tubercle, and continues distally lateral to the tibial crest (**Figure 1**) [5]. The iliotibial band is detached from its insertion using sharp dissection with a knife and reflected anteriorly and posteriorly (**Figure 2**) [5]. The interval between the IT band and the joint capsule is developed with blunt dissection, and care is taken to keep the capsule intact. As far as deep dissection is concerned, the anterior tibialis muscle is retracted posteriorly revealing the anterolateral part of proximal tibia. Consequently, the joint line is identified, and submeniscal arthrotomy is made [6]. Two or three sutures are placed in the peripheral part of the meniscus, and

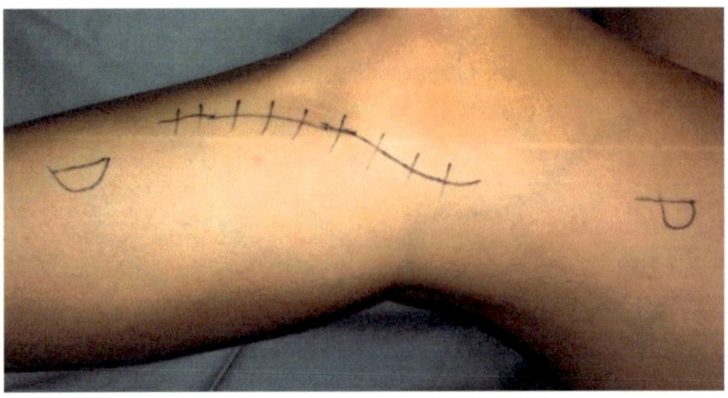

Figure 1.
Skin incision for anterolateral approach lazy "s".

retraction is applied to better visualize the articular surface. These sutures are also used to stabilize the lateral meniscus into the tibia or into the K-wire holes of the plate after fracture fixation.

According to the international literature, many orthopedic surgeons use the "straight" incision for the anterolateral approaches of tibial plateau fractures [7]. This is the second method most often used for the anterolateral approach. It consists of an incision that begins proximal to the lateral femoral epicondyle and continues distally behind Gerdy's tubercle. Depending on the fracture pattern, the skin incision can be either more posterior or anterior. Regarding superficial dissection, extensive subcutaneous soft tissue must be mobilized in order to expose the fascia of the tibialis anterior. The deep dissection that follows is the same as we describe above in "s-shaped" incision, using iliotibial band and fibula head as landmarks.

Typically, the patient is positioned in either supine or lateral decubitus position. Moreover, the patient's leg can be placed in leg-holter position for better fracture reduction due to permanent ligamentotaxis.

Structures in danger

- Short saphenous vein
- Superficial peroneal nerve
- Anterior tibial artery and deep peroneal nerve

Posterolateral plateau fractures can neither be viewed nor adequately supported with these types of procedures. Posterolateral areas cannot be visualized via the classic anterolateral approach; consequently, other techniques are needed [8]. Several osteotomies have been described for improving exposure via a standard anterolateral approach. These osteotomies help to better visualize the posterolateral part of tibial plateau and manipulate the fragments; however, it is difficult to place the adequate posterior fixation. First, the femoral epicondyle osteotomy has been used for several orthopedic surgeries, such as total knee arthroplasty or meniscal transplantation [9]. In 2015, a case report was described in which the lateral femoral epicondyle was osteotomized for better access to the posterolateral tibial plateau fracture [10]. Second, the fibula resection osteotomy has been described in 2010 and includes resection of the medial and proximal fibula. Third, the digastric fibular osteotomy has been recently described in the literature improving both the

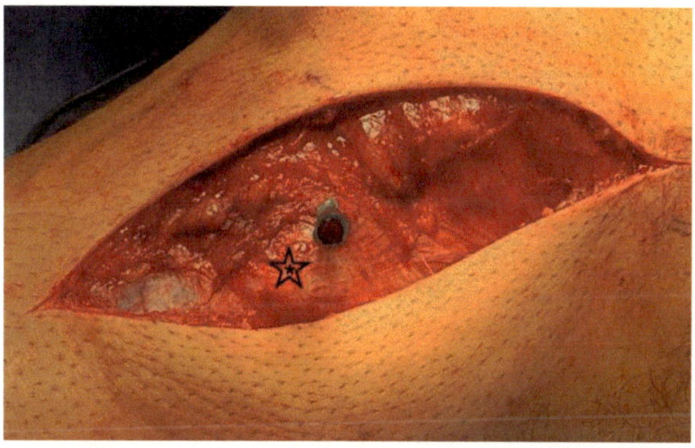

Figure 2.
Iliotibial band curved over Gerdy's tubercle.

visualization of the posterolateral articular surface and the ability to manipulate posterolateral fracture fragments.

2.2 Posterolateral approach

The posterolateral approach is ideal for the lateral tibial plateau fractures which have posterior displacement. This approach was initially described by Lobenhoffer et al. [11] in 1997 and was then modified by many surgeons such as Frosch [12] and Solomon [8] either with or without fibular osteotomy.

As Lobenhoffer [11] first described, the head of the fibula and the tibial tuberosity can be used for the orientation of the skin incision. The longitudinal cut runs laterally exactly in the middle of the distance between the tibial tuberosity and the fibula tip and has approximately 10 cm length. The peroneal nerve is identified proximal to the head of the fibula and is looped. The origin of the extensor muscle is then cut away, and the incision is continued tongue-shaped over the fibular neck. If there is a subcapital fibula fracture, this fracture is carefully mobilized. If this is not the case, a fibula osteotomy is performed after careful circumvention of the fibular neck. The origin of the extensor muscles is pushed about 1 cm distally. The meniscotibial ligament is incised, and the lateral meniscus is pulled proximally using holding threads. The fixed ligament of the tibiofibular joint is released, so that the head of the fibula can be pulled upward and back. As a result, the lateral collateral ligament relaxes and enables the lateral joint gap to be opened wide. The posterolateral tibial plateau is brought into the field of the surgeon's vision in flexion and varus as well as internal rotation. If necessary, the posterolateral tibia shaft is exposed. If extensive exposure is required, the iliotibial tract on Gerdy's tubercle can also be detached in one layer with the meniscotibial ligament.

Structures in danger

- Common peroneal nerve
- Popliteal artery
- Popliteal tendon
- Lateral superior genicular artery
- Lateral inferior genicular artery

Nowadays, a modification of the posterolateral approach is used that was described by Frosch et al. [12]. A straight incision, about 8–10 cm, is made from the medial border of the biceps femoris tendon proximally to the posteromedial part of fibula distally. Subsequently, through the skin and subcutaneous tissues, the interval between the biceps femoris tendon and the lateral gastrocnemius muscle is found. In this area, the common peroneal nerve (CPN) can be identified. In particular, it is located medial to the biceps tendon, which gives off the lateral sural cutaneous nerve (LSCN) at this level. The superficial dissection ends at the plane between lateral gastrocnemius muscle with LSCN in the lateral side and biceps femoris tendon with CPN medial. It is important to know that lateral gastrocnemius is the most medial structure in this approach. Distally, the soleus is encountered at its origin on the posterolateral tibia and fibula. Blunt elevation of the soleus will provide exposure of the proximal tibia. Moreover, the anterior tibial artery should be protected in this area, because it travels to the anterior compartment, and the common peroneal nerve. The popliteus tendon is carefully mobilized, protecting the inferolateral genicular artery from injury. Finally, submeniscus arthrotomy can be performed for better visualization of the articular surface. If more exposure is needed, transverse osteotomy of the fibular neck can be performed.

A modification of this approach was described by Solomon, with an incision along the anterior border of biceps femoris and an osteotomy of the fibula [8]. This provides the opportunity to retract the fibular head, the lateral collateral ligament, and the biceps femoris upward.

The patient may be placed in the prone, supine, or lateral decubitus position based on the patient's other injuries and the surgeon's preference.

2.3 Medial approach

The medial approach is used when an anteromedial fracture pattern of tibial plateau occurs [5]. It is difficult with this approach to obtain a good access of the articular surface without injuring the medial collateral ligament. The adductor tubercle and the medial border of the tibial crest are very important landmarks for this procedure [5].

The skin incision begins from the medial femoral epicondyle, about 2–3 cm over the joint line, and ends 2 cm posterior to the tibial crest, depending on fracture extension. The knee must be flexed about 15°–20° before proceeding with this skin incision (**Figure 3**). The superficial dissection includes the sartorius fascia, which is incised in a straight line similar to the skin. Next, the gracilis and semitendinosus

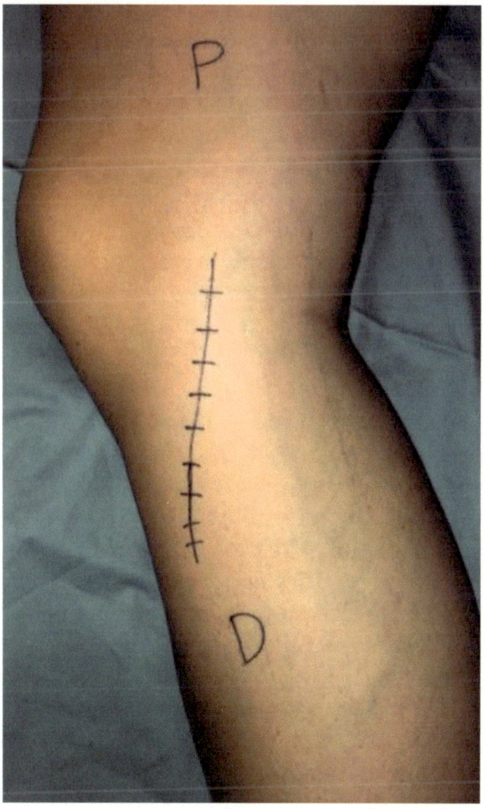

Figure 3.
Skin incision for medial approach.

tendons are identified, which arise posteriorly creating together with the sartorius the pes anserinus in the anteromedial tibia. In regard to the deep dissection, three layers exist in this area [5]. The first is the pes anserinus tendons posterior and proximal, the second is the superficial medial collateral ligament, and the third is the deep medial collateral ligament. The first and second layers can be cut off during this procedure and should be repaired after fracture fixation. The deep medial collateral can be incised by making an arthrotomy for articular surface visualization. In most cases, fracture reduction is carried out without an arthrotomy because it can be subsequently confirmed by fluoroscopic imaging.

Structures in danger

- Infrapatellar branch of saphenous nerve
- Saphenous vein
- Medial inferior genicular artery
- Popliteal artery

The patient's position is either supine with the knee flexed (~50°–60°), the ipsilateral hip external rotated and abducted or in a "leg-holter" position.

2.4 Posteromedial approach

The posteromedial approach is mainly used for shear or coronal fractures of the medial tibial plateau [13]. It is an ideal approach because it gives the opportunity to place an antiglide plate for better fixation of this type of fractures. Moreover, it can be done in either the supine or prone position. The prone position has the main advantage of being more comfortable for the surgeon. This is not recommended in dual approach strategies such as performed for concurrent lateral and medial plateau fractures, because of the need for the patient's repositioning.

In posteromedial approach in supine position [13], the surgeon should stand on the opposite side of the injured leg. The important landmarks for the incision are the medial femoral epicondyle proximal and the posterior tibial border distally. For this approach, it is important to obtain a 30° knee flexion and external rotation of the ipsilateral hip for better access of the posteromedial area. Regarding superficial dissection, the skin incision is about 8 cm, and the sartorius fascia is incised between the medial gastrocnemius posteriorly and the pes anserinus anteriorly (**Figure 4**). The saphenous nerve runs just anterior to the great saphenous vein. The medial collateral ligament lies deeper than the pes anserinus and therefore cannot be injured during this approach. The semimembranosus and the popliteus muscle insertion in the posterior tibia can be released off the bone using subperiosteal dissection for better access of the fracture area. Moreover, submeniscal arthrotomy can be done to visualize the joint directly, and sutures may be placed into the meniscus for retraction. Finally, fluoroscopic imaging is necessary to confirm the appropriate reduction of the articular surface [5].

On the other hand, the posteromedial approach in prone position was initially described in 2003 [14]. For this procedure, it is important to place a folded blanket under the ipsilateral femur allowing leg hyperextension for easier fracture reduction as mentioned by Moore. The skin incision is about 2 cm posterior and lateral than in the supine position. Its length is 8–10 cm running along the medial border of the medial gastrocnemius. The medial gastrocnemius is then

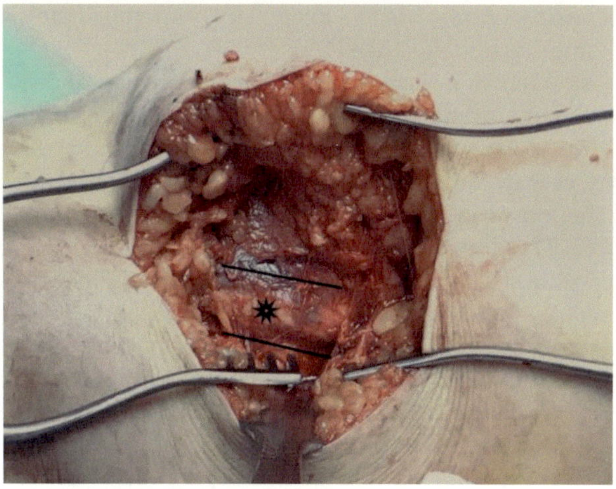

Figure 4.
The asterisk is pes anserinus tendon. Above this structure is the line for the posteromedial access between pes anserinus and medial gastrocnemius.

retracted laterally developing the interval between the medial gastrocnemius and the semimembranosus. The pes tendons are placed intact anteriorly. The deep dissection continues with the subperiosteal elevation of the popliteus muscle off its insertion in the posterolateral area of tibia. Finally, modifications of this approach exist that provide additional lateral exposure such as the "S-type" procedure [15].

Structures in danger

- Short saphenous vein
- Peroneal artery and branches
- Posterior tibial artery and nerve

2.5 Direct posterior approach

The direct posterior approach is rarely used for tibial plateau fractures. The fracture pattern treated with this approach is a shear posterior bicondylar plateau's fracture with the main fracture line in coronal plane. This method has an important disadvantage when compared to other surgical incisions, and there is a higher risk for iatrogenic injury of neurovascular structures in the popliteal fossa.

Structures in danger

- Popliteal artery
- Tibial nerve
- Sural nerve and short saphenous vein

Posterior approach was first announced in 1945 as a midline incision through popliteal fossa by Abbott and Carpenter. Many variations have been published over the years of the classic technique as "S – shape" [5], "L – type" incision [16], and lastly the "FCR"' approach to the knee [17].

An "S-shape" skin incision is made from proximal-lateral to distal-medial. In this incision, the important landmarks are the Biceps Femoris proximal, the popliteal fossa at the joint line, and the medial head of the gastrocnemius distally (**Figure 5**). We should be attentive in the superficial dissection because underneath the skin lies the lesser saphenous vein and the sural nerve, which rests immediately lateral to the vein (**Figure 6**). The deep facia is incised, and the sural nerve may be followed proximally helping the surgeon to identify the tibial nerve. The tibial nerve lies superficial and slightly lateral to the popliteal vein and artery. The popliteal fossa is recognized proximally between the medial and lateral heads of the gastrocnemius and distally between the medial border of biceps femoris and the lateral border of semimembranosus. Underneath the biceps femoris is the common peroneal nerve,

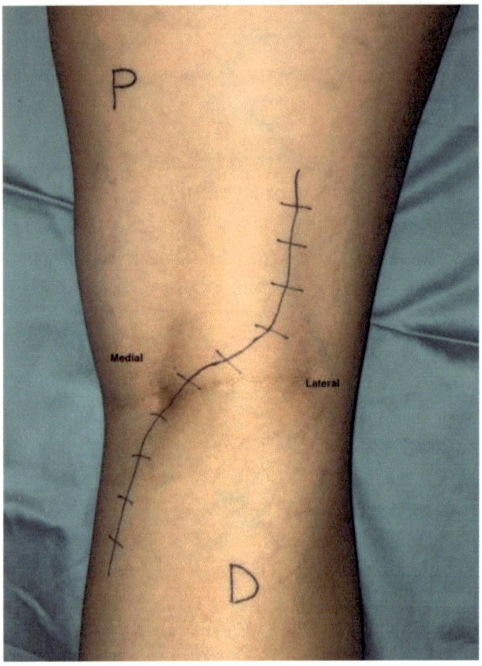

Figure 5.
Skin incision for direct posterior approach.

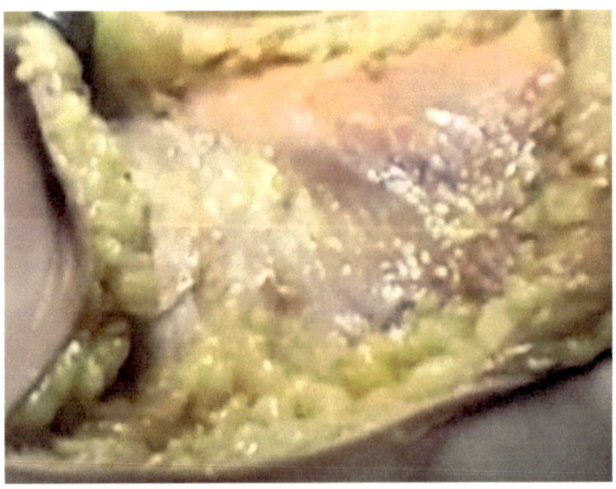

Figure 6.
The skin was mobilized and was identified the lesser saphenous vein and the sural nerve.

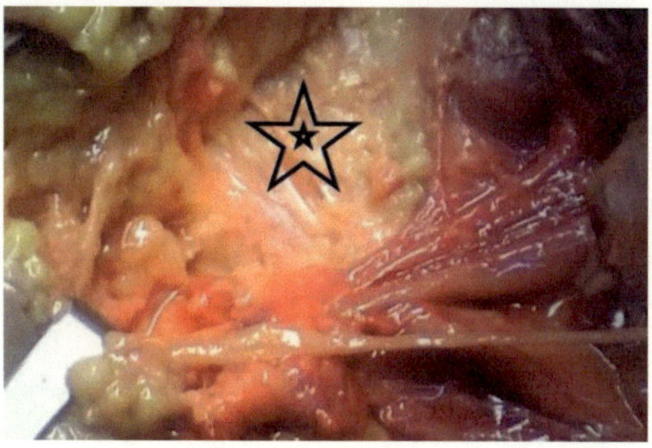

Figure 7.
The posterior capsule of knee.

which is separated from the sciatic nerve just proximal to the joint line. Depending on the fracture pattern, the deep dissection may be continued either posteromedial or posterolateral as we described above (**Figure 7**). The landmarks are Biceps femoris, the lateral and the medial gastrocnemius, and the semimembranosus tendon.

An “L-shape” incision starts superiorly and medially at the popliteus space parallel to Langer’s line. A vertical skin incision begins at the medial corner of the popliteal fossa and extends distally. Full-thickness fasciocutaneous flaps are raised protecting the sural nerve and lesser saphenous vein. The medial head of the gastrocnemius should be retracted laterally, protecting the neurovascular structures and exposing the knee capsule. The deep dissection should be done beneath the popliteus muscle in the proximal part from medial to lateral. Subsequently, the popliteus and the soleus origins are mobilized for better visualization of the posterior tibial plateau. In most cases, the entire posterior part of the tibia can be exposed without cutting the medial head of the gastrocnemius [16].

This procedure is performed with the patient in prone position and the knee slightly flexed using a bump under the ankle.

2.6 Percutaneous approach

The percutaneous approach is applied to tibial fractures with either small split of the articular surface (Schatzker I classification) or a pure depression of the lateral tibial plateau (Schatzker III classification). The incisions are about 1–2 cm in length, and fluoroscopy or arthroscopy imaging is vital for this procedure.

Percutaneous reduction should be made with a bone tamp, with percutaneous application of bone-holding forceps, and with the joystick technique and ligamentotaxis [18].

Reduction of tibial plateau fractures with small split is achieved by inserting a clamp with its ends on the lateral and medial sides, approximately 1 or 2 cm below the articular surface. The 6.5–7.3 mm cannulated screws are then placed parallel to the articular line. According to the literature, the minimal number of screws required for this procedure is three [18]. Washers are a good choice for better compressing the fracture line.

The reduction of fractures with a slight depression of the articular surface is performed by the mini-open technique. This consists of a small vertical incision on the skin (2 cm) on the lateral or medial side of the tibial metaphysis (**Figure 8**). Through this incision, a bone window is opened into the cortex, and a bone tamp is pushed for the reduction of the articulated surface (**Figure 9**). The gap that is created can be filled either with bone autografts or allografts or with calcium phosphate bone cement to support the articular surface. It is recommended to overcorrect the fracture.

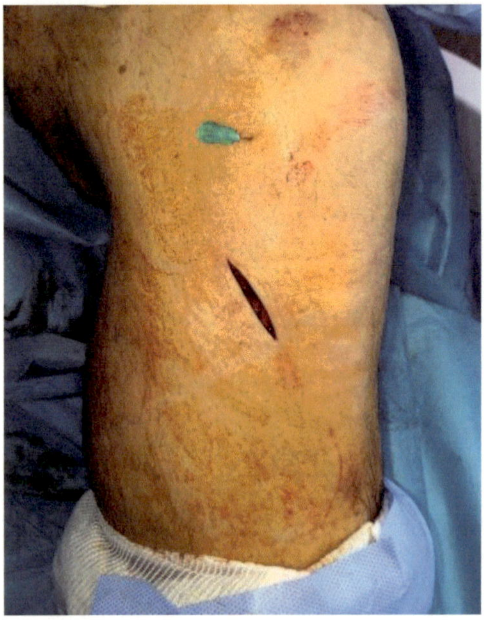

Figure 8.
Skin incision for lateral plateau fracture with percutaneous approach.

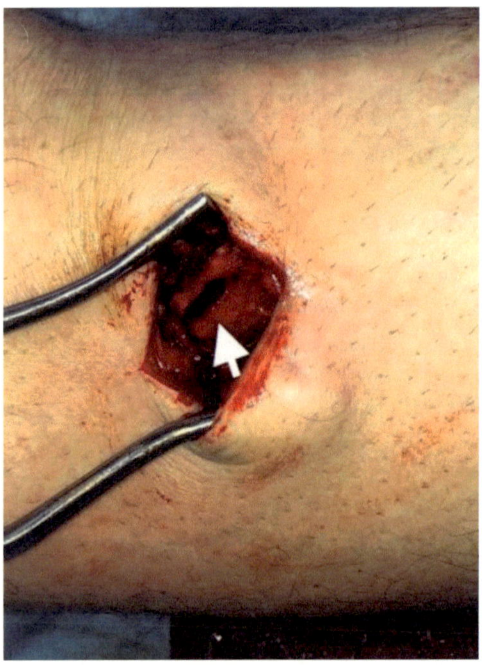

Figure 9.
Bone window in the cortex.

Radiological imaging or arthroscopic visualization of the articular surface of the tibia may be performed to evaluate adequate reduction. There are a lot of meta-analyses in the international literature, which indicate that arthroscopic fracture reduction rather than open arthrotomy achieves better functional outcomes in patients [19]. More than 10 mm of plateau depression presents an increased risk of lateral meniscus tear [20]. Therefore, slight depressed monocondylar fractures should be examined with arthroscopy after fracture reduction. It is crucial to acknowledge that knee arthroscopy can cause post-operative compartment syndrome due to fluid escaping into the tibia compartments.

Moreover, fixation plates can be used for fracture fixation, with less bone exposure. In 1989, Mast et al. [21] described the "indirect reduction" technique, thus minimizing the soft tissue damage. Subsequently, in 1997, the minimally invasive plate osteosynthesis was introduced (MIPO) by Wenda [22] and Krettek [23]. An abundance of studies followed in the international literature describes the MIPO technique and compares the advantages and disadvantages of this new method. This procedure includes small skin incisions, the application through these of the fixation plate, and furthermore percutaneous screw placing. Fracture reduction is achieved by distraction using either a distractor, a tension device, or a lamina spreader.

The main advantages of percutaneous approach and MIPO technique are risk reduction of wound complications due to minimal soft tissue damage during surgical dissection and biological fracture healing by preserving the vascularity of the bone [19]. Furthermore, this technique offers paramount benefits such as less blood loss, earlier functional rehabilitation, and shorter hospitalization [19].

3. Conclusion

Tibial plateau fractures are very common, and orthopedic surgeons should be familiar with this kind of injury. Classic surgical approaches are the lateral, the posterolateral, the medial, the posteromedial, and the direct posterior. Many variations of these techniques have been developed over the years. Nowadays, percutaneous approaches and MIPO techniques are gaining ground but only after specific indications. Before choosing the appropriate approach, it is necessary to evaluate the fracture pattern either with sufficient X-rays or CT scans.

Author details

Katsimentzas Triantafyllos[1*], Tryfon Ditsios[2*] and Kostantinos Ditsios[1*]

1 2nd Orthopaedic Department Aristotle University of Thessaloniki, G. Gennimatas Hospital, Thessaloniki, Greece

2 Medical University of Sofia, Sofia, Bulgaria

*Address all correspondence to: triantafyllos_katsimentzas@hotmail.com, tryfonditsios@gmail.com and ditsiosk@otenet.gr

References

[1] Rasmus Elsoe SEO, Larsen P, Nielsen NPH, Swenne J, Rasmussen S. Population-based epidemiology of tibial plateau fractures. Orthopedics. 2015;**38**(9):18-22

[2] Virkus WW, Berkson EM. High-energy tibial plateau fractures. The Journal of the American Academy of Orthopaedic Surgeons. 2006;**14**(1):20-31

[3] Tang HC et al. Correlation of parameters on preoperative CT images with intra-articular soft-tissue injuries in acute tibial plateau fractures: A review of 132 patients receiving ARIF. Injury. 2017;**48**(3):745-750

[4] Wasserstein D, et al. Risk of total knee arthroplasty after operatively. The Journal of Bone and Joint Surgery American. 2014;**96**:144-150

[5] Kandemir U, Maclean J. Surgical approaches for tibial plateau fractures. The Journal of Knee Surgery. 2014;**27**(1):21-29

[6] Padanilam TG, Ebraheim NA, Frogameni A. Meniscal detachment to approach lateral tibial plateau fractures. Clinical Orthopaedics and Related Research. 1995;**314**:192-198

[7] Krause M, Müller G, Frosch KH. Surgical approaches to tibial plateau fractures. Unfallchirurg. 2018;**121**(7):569-582

[8] Solomon LB, Stevenson AW, Lee YC, Baird RPV, Howie DW. Posterolateral and anterolateral approaches to unicondylar posterolateral tibial plateau fractures: A comparative study. Injury. 2013;**44**(11):1561-1568

[9] Bowers AL, Huffman GR. Lateral femoral epicondylar osteotomy: An extensile posterolateral knee approach. Clinical Orthopaedics and Related Research. 2008;**466**(7):1671-1677

[10] Yoon YC, Sim JA, Kim DH, Lee BK. Combined lateral femoral epicondylar osteotomy and a submeniscal approach for the treatment of a tibial plateau fracture involving the posterolateral quadrant. Injury. 2015;**46**(2):422-426

[11] Lobenhoffer P, Gerich T, Bertram T, Lattermann C, Pohlemann T, Tscherne H. Spezielle posteromediale und posterolaterale zugange zur versorgung von tibiakopffrakturen. Unfallchirurg. 1997;**100**(12):957-967

[12] Frosch KH, Balcarek P, Walde T, Stürmer KM. A new posterolateral approach without fibula osteotomy for the treatment of tibial plateau fractures. Journal of Orthopaedic Trauma. 2010;**24**(8):515-520

[13] Weil YA, Gardner MJ, Boraiah S, Helfet DL, Lorich DG. Posteromedial supine approach for reduction and fixation of medial and bicondylar tibial plateau fractures. Journal of Orthopaedic Trauma. 2008;**22**(5):357-362

[14] Galla M, Lobenhoffer P. Der direkte dorsale zugangsweg zur versorgung posteromedialer luxationsfrakturen des tibiakopfes. Unfallchirurg. 2003;**106**(3):241-247

[15] De Boeck H, Opdecam P. Posteromedial tibial plateau fractures: Operative treatment by posterior approach. Clinical Orthopaedics and Related Research. 1995;**320**:125-128

[16] He X et al. A posterior inverted L-shaped approach for the treatment of posterior bicondylar tibial plateau fractures. Archives of Orthopaedic and Trauma Surgery. 2013;**133**(1):23-28

[17] Berwin JT, Donovan RL, Riddick A, Kelly MB. The 'FCR' approach to the knee for the management of posterior tibial plateau fractures. Journal of

Orthopaedic Trauma. 2019 [Ahead of print]

[18] Chang HR, Yu YY, Ju LL, Le Zheng Z, Chen W, Zhang YZ. Percutaneous reduction and internal fixation for monocondylar fractures of tibial plateau: A systematic review. Orthopaedic Surgery. 2018;**10**(2):77-83

[19] Wang Y, Wang J, Tang J, Zhou F, Yang L, Wu J. Arthroscopy assisted reduction percutaneous internal fixation versus open reduction internal fixation for low energy tibia plateau fractures. Scientific Reports. 2018;**8**(1):1-9

[20] Ringus V, Lemley F, Hubbard D, Wearden S, Jones D. Lateral tibial plateau fracture depression as a predictor of lateral meniscus pathology. Orthopaedics. 2010;**33**(2):80-84

[21] Ganz R, Mast J, Jakob R, Planning and Reduction Technique in Fracture Surgery. 1989

[22] Wenda K, Runkel M, Degreif J, Rudig L. Minimally invasive plate fixation in femoral shaft fractures. Injury. 1997;**28**(Suppl 1):13-19

[23] Krettek C, Schandelmaier P, Miclau T, Tscherne H. Minimally invasive percutaneous plate osteosynthesis (MIPPO) using the DCS in proximal and distal femoral fracture. Injury. 1997;**28**(Suppl 1):20-30

Chapter 3

Midterm Results of Quality of Life after Surgical Treatment of Tibial Plateau Fractures of Type Moore V

Reiner Wirbel

Abstract

The midterm restriction of the quality of life should be evaluated and correlated with the objective radiological results in patients with the special tibial plateau fracture of type Moore V. From 2003 to 2012, 36 patients with 38 fractures were registered in a retrospective cohort study. Injury mechanism, surgical treatment, complication rate, and radiological results after a mean follow-up of 37 months and the quality of life (NRS, IKDC-form, and EQ-5D-score) after 68 months were analyzed. There were 27 men and 9 women (mean age 50.8 years) in 30 cases with high impact injury. External fixator was used in 24 cases primarily, single plate fixation was used in 12 cases, and double plate fixation was used in 25 cases. All early complication (21%) could be cured. Mean NRS was 4.53, IKDC-score was 50.46, and the EQ-5D was 7.47. The quality of life was quoted to 44% of the output value before the injury. Osteoarthritis was seen in 36 cases; severe in 19 cases and 4 requiring endoprostheses. Loss of reduction and deviation of axis were seen in 13 and 3 patients, respectively. The tibial plateau of type Moore V is a severe injury resulting in the midterm reduction of the quality of life. There is a correlation of subjective and objective results.

Keywords: dislocation-fracture, tibial plateau, result, midtem, quality of life

1. Introduction

The incidence of proximal tibial fractures shows two age peaks: on the one hand, in young patients in the third decade of life with high energy, and on the other hand, in older patients in the sixth–eighth centuries; a decade of life mostly with low-energy trauma [1–5].

Many complications regarding soft tissues such as compartment syndromes, soft tissue damage, infections are possible; their frequency is given as 10–40% [6–8], in older papers even up to 80% [9]. The long-term course affects movement restrictions, axis misalignments with a frequency of 16–27% [6–8], developing post-traumatic arthritis with up to 60% when considering the complex fractures (Schatzker V and Schatzker VI) [8] or persistent Knee instability with a frequency of 11–18% [7]. Most proximal tibial fractures require surgical therapy with the intention of restoring the articular surface and the leg axis with the option of early active and passive movement therapy to avoid joint stiffness.

Although there are some studies on the functional result achieved and the development of osteoarthritis after tibial plateau fractures [1–5, 10–16], the comparability of many studies is limited since different fracture types are often summarized.

For example, studies on the ability of skiers to do sports report that about three quarters of all patients can do sports again after tibial plateau fractures, but the level before the accident is rarely reached [17, 18]. In a study by Kraus et al. [17], only 2 out of 11 professional skiers reach their starting level after 1 year.

In addition to purely functional and objective parameters, e.g., radiological results, aspects of quality of life after surgical fracture care have been increasingly taken into account in clinical studies over the past decade. As an expression of the subjective assessment of the quality of life, so-called patient reported outcome measures (PROMs) have been established through special questionnaires. Most of these PROMs have experience in the field of endoprosthetic joint replacement [19]. Even after fracture treatment, PROMs are becoming increasingly important [20]. There are only a few studies on the quality of life after the surgical treatment of tibial plateau fractures [7, 9, 21–23]. Mostly, different fracture types with different degrees of severity are considered together.

Tibial plateau fractures are difficult to classify with little reproducibility of all classification systems [24]. In principle, plateau fractures caused by axial trauma can be differentiated from the dislocation fractures due to additional shear and rotational forces [25]. Moore distinguishes five types in his classification [25]. The term "dislocation" does not describe a knee joint dislocation here, but rather a possible accompanying injury of ligaments should be pointed out, including the injury mechanism. Type V injury ("four part") is a bicondylar fracture with a tear in the intercondylar region (**Figure 1**).

The clinical outcome after tibial plateau fractures is uncertain due to the primary damage to cartilage and subchondral bones, as well as metaphyseal compression.

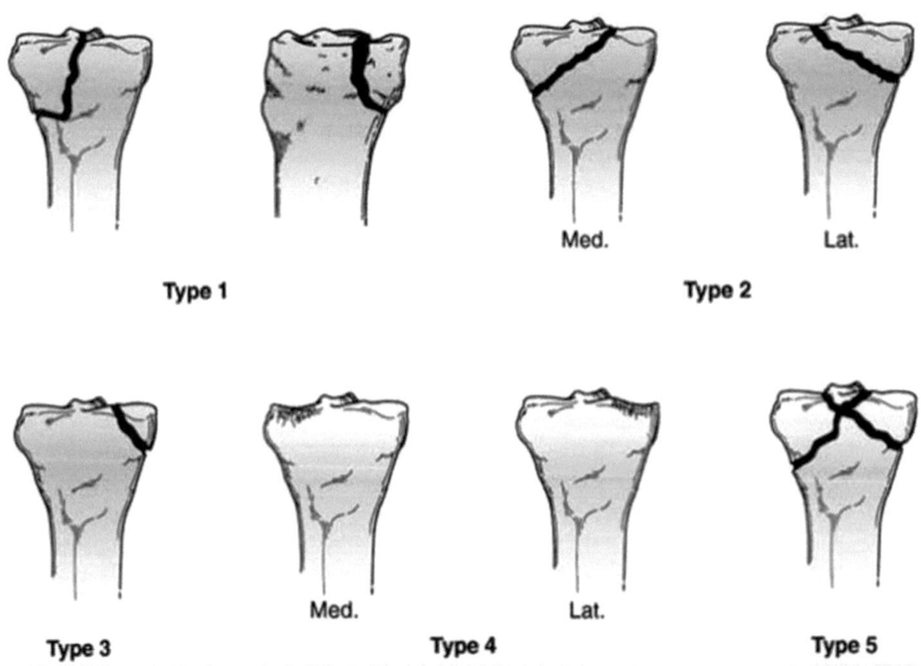

Figure 1.
Moore classification of tibial dislocation fractures.

An isolated consideration of the tibial plateau fractures of type Moore V, especially with regard to the expected quality of life, has not been available in the literature to date. For this reason, this rare special form of tibial head fracture was chosen as an expression of the most serious and complex destruction of the tibial head in the context of a multicenter survey in order to compare objectively functional clinical and radiological results with the subjectively estimated quality of life achieved.

2. Patients and methods

2.1 Patients

Patients with isolated Moore V tibial dislocation fractures on one or both sides were included. For classification, a CT examination was available preoperatively in all cases. Open fractures, fractures with accompanying vascular and/or nerve injuries as well as with accompanying fractures on the affected limb were not taken into account.

Three trauma surgery clinics took part in the multicenter retrospective cohort study, two clinics (I and II) with the mandate for maximum care and one clinic (III) as the main provider.

Over a period of 7 years (2005–2012), 193 tibial plateau fractures were treated surgically in clinic I, 25 of them were Moore V-type fractures, 20 of which were included in the study. In Clinic II, 137 tibial plateau fractures were treated surgically over a 9-year period (2003–2012). Of 10 Moore V fractures, 8 were included in the study. In Clinic III, 61 tibial head fractures were surgically stabilized over a 4-year period (2008–2012), 10 of 11 tibial head plateau fractures of the Moore V type could be checked again.

Two patients suffered bilateral fractures so that a total of 36 patients with 38 Moore V tibial plateau fractures were included in the study. The results of the patients with double-sided fractures were scored twice, each for the affected leg.

2.2 Objective parameters

In addition to the operative strategy (one-stage, two-stage care after primary fixator external treatment, and unilateral or bilateral plate osteosynthesis), the early complications within the first 2 postoperative weeks during the inpatient stay were evaluated. The last X-rays, performed on average after 37 months (range 12-102 months) after the surgery were used to determine the secondary loss of correction (misalignment, in-congruency of the tibia plateau) and the development of arthritis according to Kellgren/Lawrence [26]. The measure of the axis misalignment was determined in the whole leg.

2.3 Subjective parameters

A questionnaire after an average of 68 months (range 16–128 months) collected subjective data to assess pain, function, and quality of life, in addition to the numerical analog scale (numeric rating scale—NRS) [8, 27] for pain indication, the IKDC score (international knee documentation committee) [28], and the defined quality of life according to EQ-5D (European quality of life—5 dimensions) [29, 30].

Current pain and pain over the past 4 weeks were recorded using NRS (0–10). A total of 5 pain groups were defined: no pain: NRS = 0; mild pain: NRS = 1–3; moderate pain: NRS = 4–6; severe pain: NRS = 7–8, and very severe to severe pain: NRS = 9–10.

In addition, the ratings were collected for nightly and also divided into five groups: I: never; II: occasionally; III: every other night; IV: more often than every other night; V: every night.

The IKDC score compares the affected knee with the opposite side with regard to sporting and everyday activity, the result is given in percent (opposite side = 100%). The EQ-5D (EuroQol) questionnaire describes the five dimensions of the state of health: mobility, self-sufficiency, everyday activity, pain, and fear/depression, each with a value of 1–3. This results in total values between 5 and 15, where a low value corresponds to a high quality of life.

In addition, the numerical analogue scale (0–10) [27] was used to record the subjective assessment of the functionality of the affected knee joint, 0 being the inability to perform any normal everyday activity, possibly including sports, and 10 being the normal, excellent functionality.

2.4 Statistics

The statistical evaluation of the individual groups was carried out using the Wilcoxon rank test, and the t test for independent samples. The statistics program SPSS version 2.0 (SPSS Inc., Chicago, USA) was used for this. A p-value <0.05 was determined to be significant.

All patients were informed and gave their consent to the publication of their data.

3. Results

3.1 Patients and surgical procedures

The average age of the 36 patients was 50.8 years (range 24–74 years), that of the 27 men was 49.3 and that of the 9 women was 52 years. There were high-energy traumas in 30 cases, mostly traffic accidents and sports injuries, and only 6 cases of low-energy traumas (falls at home).

About 24 of 38 fractures were stabilized primarily on the day of the accident by external fixator. In one of these cases, the fracture healed with subsequent arthrodesis. In 12 patients, a singular, locking plate fixation was performed from lateral (4x primary, 8x secondary); in 25 patients, two plates (lateral, locking plate, dorsomedial anti-slide plate) (**Figure 2**) were applied (10x primary, 15x secondary). The anterior cruciate ligament was refixed 3 times in total; bone replacement materials (bovine cancellous bone) were only used in 4 cases.

On the day of the accident, only 4 cases were primarily openly reduced and stabilized; all other of 14 fractures were immobilized with a splint and, as in the case of secondary care after external fixation, were openly reduced and stabilized on the 4th day (range 3–7th day) on average.

3.2 Complications

In 8 patients, there were early complications within 14 days postoperatively during the inpatient stay: local infections was seen in 2 patients, implant loosening with secondary dislocation of the fracture in 4 patients, compartment syndrome in 1 patient, and infection + compartment syndrome in 1 patient. All complications could be remedied by surgical measures (debridement, vacuum sealing, refixation, and opening of the compartment). Single plate fixation was performed in seven of these complications; however, statistical significance analysis is not possible due to the small number of cases.

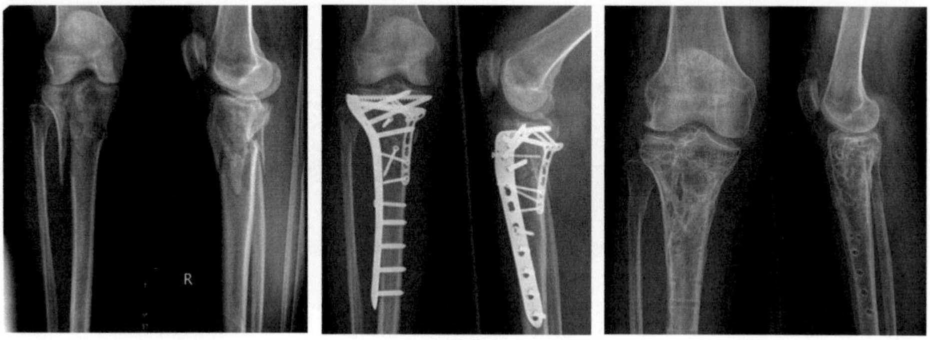

(a) (b) (c)

Figure 2.
A 58-year-old patient after falling from a chair; (a) X-ray image AP and sideways on the day of the accident; (b) postoperative; (c) 21 months later after implant removal (after 62 months: degree of osteoarthritis according to Kellgren/Lawrence 1; indication of pain NRS 0; IKDC 81.6; EQ-5D: 5).

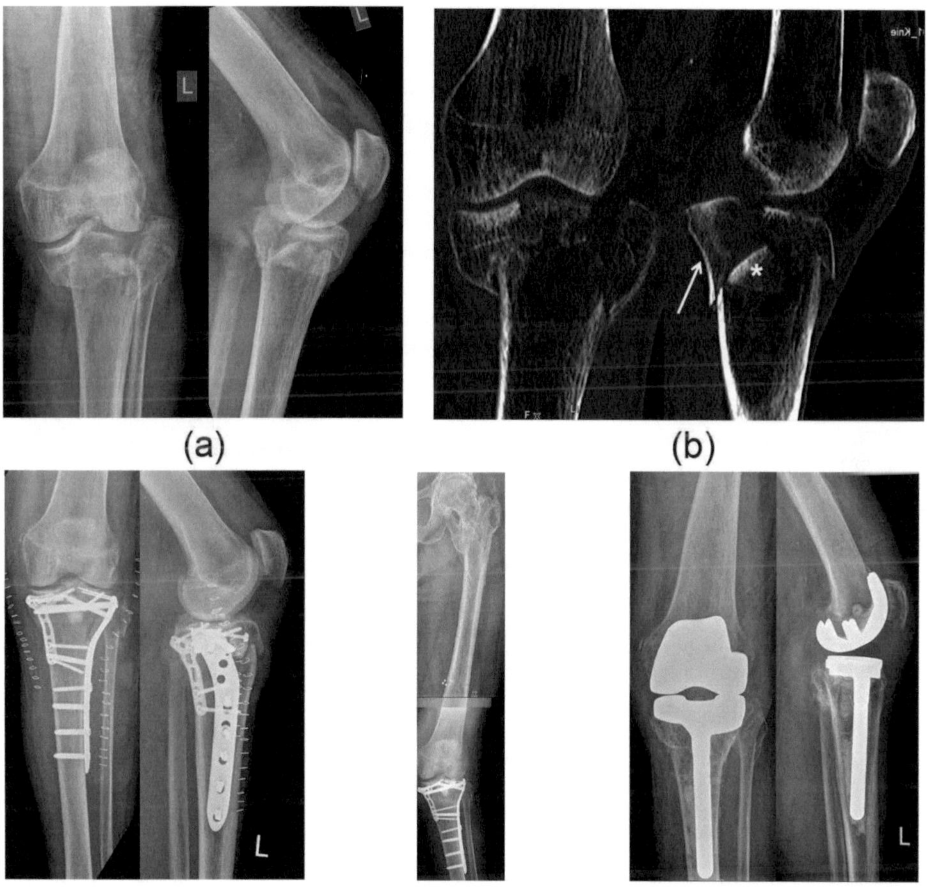

(a) (b)

(c) (d) (e)

Figure 3.
A 74-year-old patient after falling down stairs at home: (a) X-ray image AP and sideways on the day of the accident; (b) CT with coronary and sagittal incision: dorsomedial fragment (arrow), central impressed fragment (star); (c) early elective care with double plate osteosynthesis on day 3, sub-central feeding with ceramic bone substitute material; (d) CT 4 months postoperatively with evidence of lateral correction loss >2 mm and valgus position (10°); (e) early elective bicondylar surface endoprosthetic replacement due to pain and inability to walk (long tibia shaft, lateral wedge) 5 months after primary care (after 20 months: pain indication NRS 3; IKDC 52.9; EQ-5D: 6).

Kellgreen/Lawrence score*	I	II	III	IV
n	1	13	16	3
Ø NRS pain [0–10]	0	4.38	5.4	6.3
Loss of correction**	bis < 2 mm		≥2 mm	
n	24		13	
Ø NRS pain [0–10]	3.88		5.42 [p = 0.04]	
Ø pain at night [1–5]	1.88		3 [p = 0.03]	

**n = 33—4 patients with secondary endoprosthesis and 1 patient with arthrodesis were not evaluated.*
***n = 37—the patient with arthrodesis was excluded.*

Table 1.
Relationship between pain and degree of arthritis and loss of correction in patients with tibial plateau fractures of the type Moore V.

3.3 Objective results

Since a patient was treated in the external fixator with subsequent arthrodesis, a fracture loss in the 37 of the 38 fractures could be recorded in the average 37 months postoperative X-rays: 1 mm in 10 cases, 2 mm in 7 cases, and >2 mm in 6 cases. In 2 patients, there was a valgus deformity (in 1 patient 10° and in 1 patient >20°), and in 1 patient, a varus deformity (10°). A secondary correction loss of ≥2 mm (**Figure 3d**) was shown in 8 patients in the group of bilateral plate fixation (43%) and in 5 patients in the group of single plate fixation (57%). In view of the small number of cases, a significant statistical difference cannot be obtained here either. Endoprosthetic joint replacement was performed in 4 patients after an average of 6 months (range 5–8 months). Except for one case with a necessary proximal tibia replacement over 6 cm, bicondylar surface replacement endoprostheses were used (**Figure 3e**).

One patient was healed in the external fixator with primary arthrodesis. In 5 of the remaining 33 patients, an implant removal was removed after an average of 19.8 months (range 3–54 months).

Radiologically, all 33 remaining fractures showed signs of arthritis after an average of 37 months. According to Kellgren and Laurence, the degrees of severity were distributed as follows: grade I: n = 1 (**Figure 2**); grade 2: n = 13; grade 3: n = 16; and grade 4: n = 3 (**Table 1**).

At the time of the survey, 4 patients (10.5%) had partial disability assessment or a corresponding application due to the knee injury.

4. Subjective results

4.1 Pain and swelling

Within the last 4 weeks before the survey, only 2 patients stated that they had no pain. The division of pain sensation into 5 groups and the nocturnal pain indication are shown in **Figure 4**. On average, the NRS (0–10) for the pain in the last 4 weeks was 5.25 and for the night pain (1–5) was 2.27.

There was no influence from the primary surgical procedure (one, two, unilateral, and bilateral plate fixation). The mean pain reported during the past 4 weeks was higher in patients with a correction loss ≥2 mm (NRS 5.42) than in patients without loss of correction (NRS 3.88). The difference was statistically significant

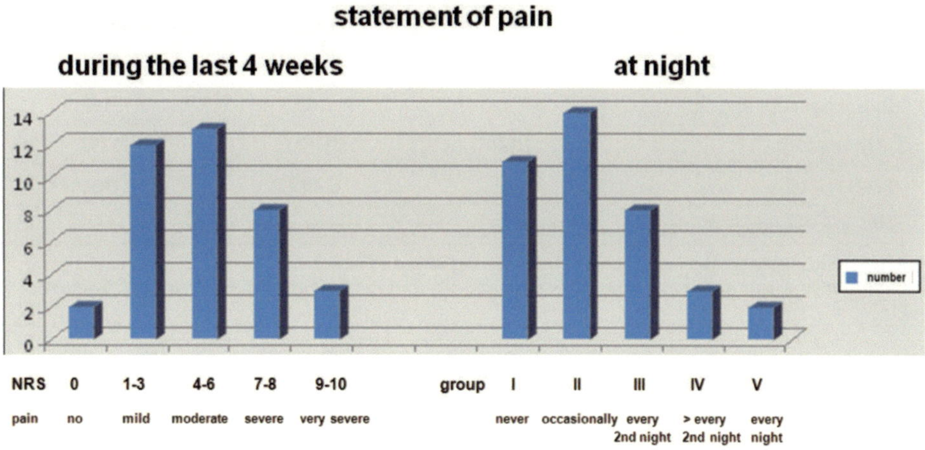

Figure 4.
Pain sensation in 36 patients with 38 tibial plateau fractures of the type Moore V (2 patients with bilateral fractures scored twice, each for the affected knee).

(p = 0.04). With regard to the nocturnal pain indication, this difference (NRS 3 versus 1.88) was also significant (p = 0.03).

With regard to the assessment of the tendency to swell during the last 4 weeks before the survey in 5 degrees of severity, similar distributions resulted as with the pain indication: "not at all" was reported by 5 patients, "somewhat" by 21 patients, "fairly" by 8 patients, "very" by 3 patients, and "extremely" was reported by 1 patient.

4.2 Sports and everyday activity

Similar results were found in the survey on sporting and everyday activities. Only 1 patient reaches the highest activity level (soccer); moderate activity (running) was possible in 6 patients; light activity (walking) was possible in 25 patients; and no sporting activity was possible in 6 patients.

Very strenuous everyday activities were only given in one case, strenuous in 4, moderately strenuous in 7, light activities in 27, and no activities in 3 cases.

4.3 IKDC and ED-5Q scores

The mean for the IKDC score was 50.46 (range 25.3–93.1). There were no significant differences regarding the operative strategy (one, two, unilateral, and bilateral plate fixation), gender or the fact of a secondary loss of correction. In the group of patients who had complications, the value was reduced compared to the group without complications (42 versus 52), but the difference was not significant. The 4 patients who received or applied for an invalidity pension showed a significantly poorer IKDC score compared to the group without any relief (41.25 versus 51.56, p = 0.01).

The mean of the EQ-5D score was 7.47 (range 5–10; standard deviation 1.5). The results were better in female patients when there was no complication or secondary correction loss; however, the differences were not all significant. When retiring or applying for a pension, the EQ-5D score was 8.5 and without retirement it was 7.35 (p = 0.016).

	Median (ø)	Range	Standard deviation
NRS pain* [0–10]	5.25	0–10	±2.5
Pain at night** [1–5]	2.27	1–5	±1.6
IKDC [0–100]	50.46	25.3–93.1	±17.57
EQ-5D [5–15]	7.47	5–10	±1.5
NRS functionality [0–10]	4.53	0–9	±2.61

**Pain reported during the last 4 weeks before the questioning after ø 68 months.*
***Classification of pain at night: 1—never; 2—occasionally; 3—every 2nd night; 4—>every 2nd night; 5—every night.*

Table 2.
Parameters to determine the quality of life in 36 patients with 38 tibial plateau fractures of the type Moore V.

4.4 Functionality

According to the NRS, the mean value for the affected knee before the injury was 9.68 (range 6–10, standard deviation 0.904) and at the time of the survey was 4.53 (range 0–7, standard deviation 2.617). The difference was significant ($p < 0.001$). The NRS was significantly ($p = 0.019$) lower in patients with complications (2.63) compared to those without complications (5.03). There was also a tendency toward lower values in patients with a correction loss ≥2 mm and patients who received a disability pension or applied for it, but these differences were not significant. The information on the subjective indication of pain, the IKDC score, the ED-5D score, and the functionality of the affected knee joint are listed in **Table 2**. There were no other differences with regard to the surgical procedure or the surgical strategy.

5. Relationship between objective and subjective results

The degree of arthritis correlated with the pain information (**Table 1**). Only 1 patient showed a Kellgren/Lawrence grade 1 (**Figure 2**) with a pain indication of NRS = 0. An arthritis of grade 2 correlated with an average NRS of 4.38 (range 3–8), an arthritis of grade 3 with an NRS of 5.4 (range 2–10), and an arthritis of grade 4 with an NRS of 6.3 (range 5–8); there was no statistical significance.

When all parameters were considered, the quality of life after tibial plateau fractures of the type Moore V was reduced to 44% of their initial value.

6. Discussion

Tibial plateau fractures are rare and they make up about 1–2% of all bone injuries [1–5]. Approximately 80–85% are plateau fractures and approximately 15–20% are "dislocation fractures" [25]. The most serious form of dislocation fracture, the type V fracture according to Moore, is still considered difficult to treat with an unfavorable prognosis. Depending on the soft tissue situation, the two-stage procedure is preferred for the operative care. After primary immobilization in the joint fixator, the treatment algorithm includes external and necessary CT diagnostics for precise fracture analysis, the definitive osteosynthesis after 5–6 days; angle-stable mono- or bicondylar plate osteosynthesis are usually performed [1–5, 7, 10–16, 21–23, 31]. The dorsomedial fragment, which has a certain key function due to the generally intact side band, is to be stabilized with an anti-slide plate [1–3, 10, 12, 14, 16, 31].

It was striking in our own case series that bone replacement materials were only used in 4 cases (10.5%). In the literature, this requirement is stated to be around 30% [1–5]. This discrepancy can be caused by the selected fracture type (Moore V); the defect zone is usually filled in with plateau fractures of the impression type.

Clinical-functional and radiological results after tibial plateau fractures have been described several times, but mostly different types of fractures are summarized. The follow-up rate is often only 50–60% [14, 31]. In our study, all patients could be asked about their quality of life with a targeted questionnaire. The follow-up period of 5.6 years is in the average range compared to the literature.

The average age in our study is 50.8 years lower than in most other studies. The reason for this may be that tibial head dislocation fractures of the Moore V type were considered separately. This usually requires high-energy trauma, in the study presented in 30 out of 36 patients, to whom younger patients are increasingly exposed. However, even older patients may experience a tibial plateau fracture of type Moore V due to their possible reduced bone quality in the context of low-energy trauma. This does not change the operational care strategy of the two-stage approach given above.

The complication rates after surgical treatment when considering all tibial plateau fractures fluctuate between 2 and 40% [6, 9], when isolating type C fractures according to the AO classification up to 40% complications are reported [10, 12, 14, 16, 21, 31]. Local infections and implant loosening are summarized. In the study presented, this value was 21.1%. In an older study, infection rates of 32% for unilateral plate fixation and even 82% for bilateral plate fixation are given [9]. However, this information can only be used to a limited extent, and 47 tibia head fractures were taken into account. Double plate fixation was only used in 8 out of 24 type C fractures, with local infection or wound healing impairment occurring in 7 cases. By recognizing the importance of soft tissue protection, this high infection rate could also be reduced by developing minimally invasive approaches, especially on the medial tibia head [6]. Extended medial approaches have also been described to address this important medio-dorsal fragment [32].

The discrepancy in the number of uni- (in 12 cases) and bilateral plate fixation (in 25 cases) in the study presented for the same fracture type could be explained by the fact that different surgeons at different clinics were at risk despite the knowledge of a better radiological outcome due to the local soft tissue situation of an infection had foregone an additional medial plate system.

Various authors generally describe a higher secondary correction loss of up to 15% after lateral plate fixation alone [16, 31]. This could not be confirmed in our own case series; however, the number of cases was too small to make a statistical statement here.

The frequency of secondary axis misalignments is different in the literature, mostly given as 10–30% [1–5, 16, 22, 31]. In our own approach, 3 axis deviations (7.8%) were seen, whereby only misalignments of >10° were taken into account. The consideration of an axis deviation "only" from 10° can be cited as a weakness of the study. Smaller deviations have also been measured in various studies [6–8]. The limitation described was justified because clinical relevance with the possible indication for correction often only arises from a deviation of >10°. However, this cannot rule out that even minor axis deviations can have consequences for the functional outcome.

There is no precise information in the literature about the incidence of necessary secondary endoprosthetic replacement. In the presented study, 4 endoprostheses (10.5%) were necessary in the course. Primary endoprosthetic replacement has not been of any importance, at least to date, for the form of fracture presented. The quality of reduction, i.e., continuous restoration of the articular surface and alignment of the axis correlates with the clinical outcome in most, both older [33–35] and younger [1–5, 8, 10–16, 36] publications. In the work by Marsh et al. [37], however, there are no reliable indications that a continuous restoration of the joint surface really affects the overall clinical result.

A big problem of many of these studies is again listed here that different fracture types are combined.

The success of therapy must be assessed more than ever by the patient himself. In addition, the patient reported outcome measures (PROMs) already established in endoprosthetic replacements are becoming increasingly important in fracture care [17, 18].

Studies about the quality of life of tibial plateau fractures are rare. For example, Rossbach et al. [7] reported in a recently published study on the quality of life and work ability of 41 patients with surgically treated tibial plateau fractures. A total of 18 fractures were classified as C fractures according to the AO classification, 11 as dislocation fractures according to the Moore classification, of which only 2 were type V fractures. Since there were also many multiple injuries, it could not be determined exactly whether the restriction of the SF-36 score was solely due to the tibial fracture. Overall, however, there was also a significant correlation between the radiological result and the quality of life achieved. This could also be confirmed in our case series with a correlation between pain information and degree of activity of the arthritis or secondary loss of correction (**Table 2**). The correlation was even significant with regard to the last parameter. However, given the small number of cases, this correlation is only favored as a trend.

Overall, the data of the subjective pain assessment in the own case series are worse than in the comparative literature [7, 11, 21–23]. Only 5% of our patients said they had no pain and 25% experienced severe to very severe pain. Two phenomena can be responsible for this. On the one hand, only the severe form of the type Moore—V fracture is considered in the presented study; most of the other studies also include other forms of fracture. On the other hand, the patient age is lower. Younger patients tend to idealize their state of health before the injury and are generally more demanding than older patients, with poorer results.

Similar results can be seen for the assessment of the function of the affected knee joint and the activity level of the patients, recorded using the IKDC score. The results correlate with the information provided by Jansen et al. [10], which examined 22 patients with 23 type C fractures (AO classification) with an average follow-up of 67 months. Only 3 patients (13.6%) had a good to very good result in the IKDC score, and 14 patients (60%) had a low activity level. The follow-up period is almost identical to that of your own case series.

The assessment of sporting activity as a measure of the level of activity achieved and the quality of life shows similar results. Only 1 of the 36 patients (2.7%) achieved the highest level of activity (football); only slight activity (walking) was possible in 25 patients (69.4%) and no activity was possible in 6 patients (16.6%). This can also clarify the severity of the injury. In the literature, a return to sporting activity is reported at a lower level in about 75% of patients when all tibial plateau fractures are considered. However, high-performance athletes rarely reach their starting level despite intensive training [17]. In a study by Loibl et al. 62% of recreational athletes with intra-articular tibial plateau fractures rated their sporting activity level after 7 years on average as similar as before the accident, while 38% rated this as significantly worse [18]. The worse values in our patient series can be explained by the isolated consideration of the Moore V fractures.

With regard to the development of arthritis, there were differences in the patient's own case series compared to the information provided by Jansen et al. [10]. Missing signs of arthritis were only found in 3% of our own study. Jansen et al. saw in 30% and severe signs of osteoarthritis in 59% and 26%. The discrepancy could again be due to the fact that the heavy form of the Moore V fracture was considered in isolation.

Altogether, the tibial plateau fracture of type Moore V represents a serious injury; the patient's quality of life is considered to be 44% of their original value after an average of 5 years after considering all parameters. The subjective information on quality of life correlates with the objective radiological parameters (degree of arthritis and loss of correction).

In a recently published clinical study [38], a reduction in the quality of life to 75 was observed in 71 patients with tibial plateau fractures after 1 year. However, all fracture types were taken into account; a connection between radiological osteoarthritis development and functional outcome could not be demonstrated.

A significant limitation of the presented study could be seen in the fact that the subjective information was collected after an average of 68 months, whereas the objective radiological criteria were obtained after an average of 37 months. The information in the study by Rademakers et al. [2] confirm, however, that if 109 tibial plateau fractures are considered over a follow-up period of up to 27 years, a significant improvement in knee joint function can no longer be expected after more than a year. Since there was no current radiological diagnosis at the time of the examination, even stronger and more frequent signs of arthritis may have been added in the meantime.

It can also be critically noted that the secondary loss of correction was measured using a native X-ray examination. A CT examination would have given more precise data with a possibly higher incidence of joint levels or mismatches of the articular surfaces.

Therefore, as with the further point of criticism of the small number of cases, the information on the relationship between quality of life and radiological result can only be interpreted or understood as tendencies.

Tibial plateau fractures of the type Moore V are severe injuries of the knee joint with a clearly limited quality of life in the medium term, whereby their subjective assessments correlate with the objective radiological parameters.

Therefore, the surgical treatment of tibial plateau fractures must be as precise as possible, i.e., to strive for step-free reconstruction of the articular surface and the tibial shaft axis.

Author details

Reiner Wirbel
Department of Trauma-, Hand- and Reconstructive Surgery, Verbundkrankenhaus Bernkastel-Wittlich, Wittlich, Germany

*Address all correspondence to: reiner.wirbel@web.de

References

[1] Biggi F, Fabio S, D'Antimo C, et al. Tibial plateau fractures: Internal fixation with locking plates and the MIPO technique. Injury. 2010;**41**: 1178-1182

[2] Rademakers MV, Kerkhoffs GM, Sierevelt IN, et al. Operative treatment of 109 tibial plateau fractures: Five- to 27-year follow-up results. Journal of Orthopaedic Trauma. 2007;**21**:5-10

[3] Musahl V, Tarkin I, Kobbe P, et al. New trends and techniques in open reduction and internal fixation of fractures of the tibial plateau. Journal of Bone and Joint Surgery. 2009;**91-B**:426-433

[4] Weigel DP, Marsh J. High-energy fractures of the tibial plateau. Knee function after longer follow-up. Journal of Bone and Joint Surgery. 2002;**84-A**:1541-1551

[5] Stevens DG, Beharry R, McKee MD. The long-term functional outcome of operatively treated tibial plateau fractures. Journal of Orthopaedic Trauma. 2001;**15**:312-320

[6] Papagelopoulos PJ, Partsinevelos AA, Themistocleous GS, et al. Complications after tibial plateau fracture surgery. Injury. 2006;**37**:475-484

[7] Rossbach BP, Faymonville C, Muller LP et al. Quality of life and ability to work after surgical treatment of tibial head fractures. Unfallchirurg. 2016;**119**:27-35

[8] Manidakis N, Dosani A, Dimitriou R, et al. Tibial plateau fractures: Functional outcome and incidence of osteoarthritis in 125 cases. International Orthopaedics. 2010;**34**:565-570

[9] Young MJ, Barrack RL. Complications of internal fixation of tibial plateau fractures. Orthopaedic Review. 1994;**23**:149-154

[10] Jansen H, Frey SP, Doht S, et al. Midterm results after complex intra-articular fractures of the tibial plateau. Journal of Orthopaedic Science. 2013;**18**:569-577

[11] Timmers TK, van der Ven DJ, de Vries LS, et al. Functional outcome after tibial plateau fracture osteosynthesis: A mean follow-up of 6 years. The Knee. 2014;**21**:1210-1215

[12] Yao Y, Lv H, Zan J, et al. Functional outcome of bicondylar tibial plateau fractures treated with dual buttress plates and risk factors: A case series. Injury. 2014;**45**:1980-1984

[13] Vasanad GH, Antin SM, Akkimaradi RC, et al. Surgical management of tibial plateau fractures—A clinical study. Journal of Clinical and Diagnostic Research. 2013;**12**:3128-3130

[14] Prasad GT, Kumar TS, Kumar RK, et al. Functional outcome of Schatzker type V and VI tibial plateau fractures treated with dual plates. Indian Journal of Orthopaedics. 2013;**47**:188-194

[15] Gaston P, Will EM, Keatin JF. Recovery of knee function following fracture ofthe tibial platcau. Journal of Bone and Joint Surgery. 2005;**87-B**:1233-1236

[16] Egol KA, Su E, Tejwani NC, et al. Treatment of complex tibial plateau fractures using the less invasive stabilization system plate: Clinical experience and a laboratory comparison with double plating. The Journal of Trauma. 2004;**57**:340-346

[17] Kraus TM, Martetschläger F, Müller D, et al. Return to sports activity after tibial plateau fractures: 89 cases with minimum 24-month follow-up. Journal of Sports Medicine. 2012;**40**:2845-2852

[18] Loibl M, Bäumlein M, Massen F, et al. Sports activity after surgical treatment of intra-articular tibial plateau fractures in skiers. Journal of Sports Medicine. 2013;**41**:1340-1347

[19] Baker PN, Beekan DJ, Lees, et al. The effect of surgical factors on early patient-reported outcome measures (PROMS) following total knee replacement. Journal of Bone and Joint Surgery. 2012;**94-B**:1058-1066

[20] Hutchings L, Fox R, Chesser T. Proximal femoral fractures in the elderly: How are we measuring outcome? Injury. 2011;**42**:1205-1213

[21] Ahearn N, Oppy A, Haliday R. The outcome following fixation of bicondylar tibial plateau fractures. The Bone and Joint Journal. 2014;**96-B**:956-962

[22] Persiani P, Gurzi MD, Di Domenica M, et al. Risk analysis in tibial plateau fractures: Association between severity, treatment and clinical outcome. Musculoskeletal Surgery. 2013;**97**:131-136

[23] Dattani R, Slobogean GB, O'Brien PJ, et al. Psychometric analysis of measuring functional outcomes in tibial plateau fractures using the short form (SF-36), short musculoskeletal functions assessment (SMFA) and the Western Ontario McMaster osteoarthritis (WOMAC) questionnaires. Injury. 2013;**44**:825-829

[24] Gicquel T, Najihi N, Vendeuvre T, et al. Tibial plateau fractures: Reproducibility of three classifications (Schatzker, AO, Duparc) and a revised Duparc classification. Orthopaedics & Traumatology, Surgery & Research. 2013;**99**:805-816

[25] Moore TM. Fracture-dislocation of the knee, section II, general orthopedics. Clinical Orthopaedics and Related Research. 1981;**156**:128-140

[26] Kellgren JH, Lawrence JS. Radiological assessment of osteoarthritis. Annals of the Rheumatic Diseases. 1957;**16**:494-501

[27] Westhoff G. Handbook of Psychosocial Measuring Instruments—A Compendium for Epidemiological and Clinical Research on Chronic Disease. Göttingen: Hogrefe; 1993

[28] Mistake JJ, Anderson AF, Boland AL, et al. Development and validation of the international knee documentation committee subjective knee form. The American Journal of Sports Medicine. 2001;**69**:600-613

[29] Rabin R, de Charro F. ED-5D: A measure of health status from the EuroQol group. Annals of Medicine. 2001;**33**:337-343

[30] Brooks R. EuroQol: The current state of play. Health Policy. 1996;**37**:53-72

[31] Gosling T, Schandelmaier P, Müller M, et al. Single lateral locked screw plating of bicondylar tibial plateau fractures. Clinical Orthopaedics and Related Research. 2005;**439**:207-214

[32] Potocnik P, Acklin YP, Sommer C. Operative strategy in postero-medial fracture-dislocation of the proximal tibia. Injury. 2011;**42**:1060-1065

[33] Vanderberghe D, Cuypers L, Rombouts L, et al. Internal fixation of tibial plateau fractures using the AO instrumentation. Acta Orthopaedica Belgica. 1990;**56**:431-442

[34] Burri C, Bartzke G, Coldewey J, et al. Fractures of the tibial plateau. Clinical Orthopaedics and Related Research. 1979;**138**:84-93

[35] Lansinger O, Bergman B, Korner L, et al. Tibial condylar fractures: A twenty-year follow-up. The Journal of Bone and Joint Surgery. 1986;**68-A**:13-19

[36] Conserva V, Vincenti G, Allegretti G, et al. Retrospective review of tibial plateau fractures by two methods without staging. Injury. 2015;**46**:1951-1956

[37] Marsh JL, Buckwalter J, Gelberman R, et al. Articular fractures: Does an anatomic reduction really change the result? The Journal of Bone and Joint Surgery. 2002;**84-A**:1259-1271

[38] van Dreumel RL, van Wunnik BP, Janssen L, et al. Mid- to long-term functional outcome after open reduction and internal fixation of tibial plateau fractures. Injury. 2015;**46**:1608-1612

Section 2

Non-Articular Tibia Fractures

Chapter 4

Far Proximal and Far Distal Tibial Fractures: Management with Intramedullary Nails

Luis Bahamonde, Alvaro Zamorano and Pierluca Zecchetto

Abstract

Operative treatment of tibial fractures located at the proximal metaphyseal-epiphyseal and distal metaphyseal-epiphyseal areas, including those with articular extensions, is a technical challenge. Common methods for surgical management include plates (locking and nonlocking), external fixation devices, and intramedullary nails. All these methods have shown satisfactory results in terms of quality of reduction and clinical and radiological outcomes. The authors present some technical methods and strategies that have been useful for the surgical approach, reduction, and fixation of these lesions with the use of locked nails.

Keywords: proximal, distal tibial fractures

1. Introduction

Tibial fractures located in the proximal and distal meta-epiphyseal areas pose a technical challenge for surgical management [1, 2]. A very proximal or distal fracture fragment, which may include intraarticular involvement, is difficult for proper reduction and alignment with the diaphysis [3], and at times, there is little bone stock available for solid fixation, either with plates or with nails. Aside from this, the soft tissue envelope is tenuous – especially at the distal tibia – and may result in damage due to trauma [4]. The evaluation of the quality of soft tissues is key when selecting any method for surgical treatment. Common surgical techniques include plates (either locking or nonlocking), locked intramedullary nails, and external fixators [5, 6]. These methods have shown good results in terms of quality of reduction and functional outcomes.

Intramedullary nailing (extreme nailing) is a competent method for the management of these difficult injuries [1]. Careful planning and surgical technique are essential for good reduction and stable fixation [7]. The authors present some strategies, technical considerations, and methods that have been useful for the achievement of these goals.

2. General preparation and positioning

Positioning of the patient is the first and at the same time critical aspect to be considered that influences the final surgical result. For conventional, transpatellar or parapatellar intramedullary nailing, the senior author (LB) uses a thigh holder

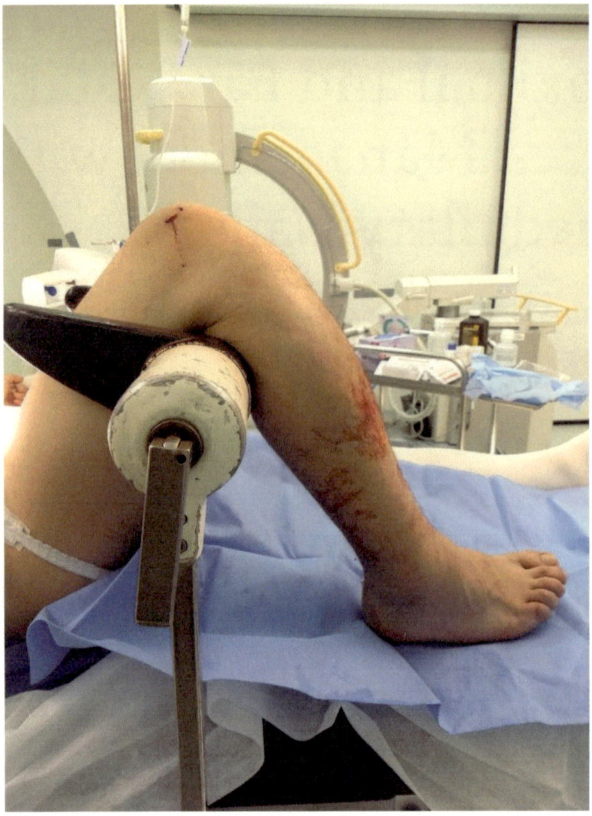

Figure 1.
The position for conventional transpatellar approach. The use of a thigh holder allows for knee flexion greater than 90°, facilitating approach, reduction, and nail insertion in most tibial fractures. For more proximal injuries, the proximal fragment can be pushed manually in further flexion for proper alignment and reduction.

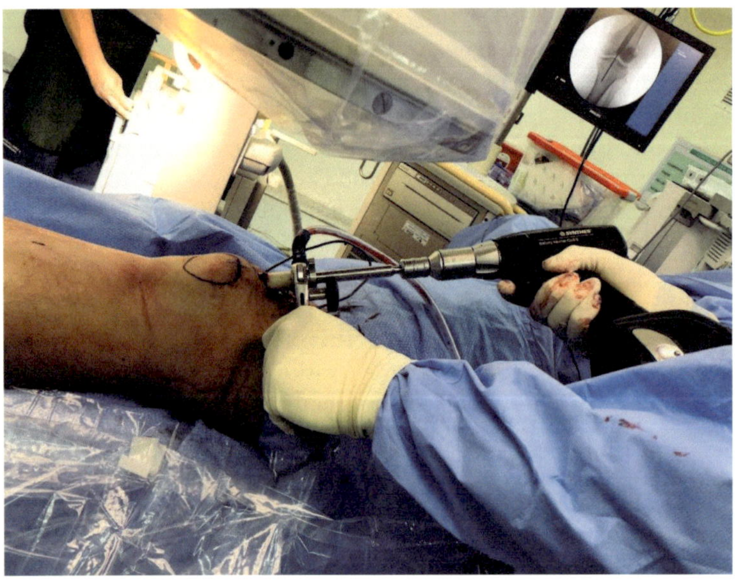

Figure 2.
Intraoperative photography showing the different elements necessary for proper suprapatellar insertion technique: special instrumentation and continuous verification of the procedure by fluoroscopy.

that is commonly utilized for arthroscopic procedures. It is located at the level of the popliteal space or just proximal to it, allowing a knee flexion of 90° or more, and with the foot barely touching the operating table (**Figure 1**). This facilitates exposure of the entry point and an easy insertion of the intramedullary guide and the nail. The transpatellar approach allows direct visualization and palpation of the correct entry point, so intraoperative X-rays are regularly not needed for this step [8, 9].

The more novel suprapatellar approach is done with the knee in a semi-extended position, for which a pad or small roller is located at the level of the popliteal space. This technique requires special instrumentation (**Figure 2**). Aside from this, clear AP and lateral X-ray views of the proper entry point are important [10]. Although there is not a clearly proven advantage over the traditional transpatellar approach, the simplicity of the leg positioning has made it much more popular [11].

3. Intramedullary nailing of far-proximal tibial fractures

Very proximal tibial fractures, which may include a simple articular split or depression fracture of one or both plateaus, are suitable for intramedullary fixation. Planning should consider the energy involved and "personality" of the fracture (open or closed fractures, concomitant injuries, damage to soft tissues, displacement of bone fragments, articular involvement, and quality of bone stock in the proximal fragment) [12].

Roughly, even with modern methods for improving intraoperative reduction, malalignment remains up to 10% of the cases. Three factors should be taken into account to prevent malalignment: first, there is a natural tendency for the proximal fragment to hyperextend as the knee flexes, due to the pull of the patellar tendon. Second, valgus deformity also may occur, usually due to a combination of soft-tissue pull and misplacement of the starting point for nail insertion. The anatomy of the triangular-shaped proximal tibia and diaphysis causes the medullary canal to be aligned in correspondence to a point slightly lateral to the midline of the epiphysis. Third, the nail design, in particular, is the so-called Herzog angle. If this angle is at the level or distal to the fracture, it tends to displace posteriorly the distal fragment.

For most surgeons, the optimal starting point is proximal to the anterior edge of the articular margin and slightly medial to the lateral tibial spine [10].

In conjunction with careful selection of a correct starting point, we utilize three methods to aid in proper reduction and counteract deformity forces: a suprapatellar approach with the leg in a semi-extended position [13], limited open reduction and provisional fixation with one or two one-third 3.5 mm plates [10], and the use of blocking (poller) screws to direct the path of the nail and facilitate proper reduction [14].

- Suprapatellar approach and semi-extended positioning: for this, a regular radiolucent table suffices. A radiolucent pad or roller is held under the knee of the affected extremity with 10 or 20° of knee flexion, which is maintained during the procedure. The semi-extended position allows easy alignment of the proximal fragment with the diaphysis by neutralizing patellar tendon pull. It also results very useful for expeditious reduction and nailing of distal fractures and facilitates intraoperative fluoroscopy (**Figure 2**). As cited before, special instrumentation is required, and careful selection of the entry point and initial trajectory of the guide must be verified [10, 13].

- Direct reduction with small plates: a limited direct approach of the fracture site is performed, and one or two orthogonal 3.5 mm third-tubular plates are inserted to maintain proper fracture reduction and counteracting deforming forces. Most of the times, large cortical fragments are present, proximally and distally, which allow restoration of adequate alignment between the main components of the fracture (**Figure 3**). Variable degrees of knee flexion can be therefore managed without losing reduction. As such, conventional nail insertion through a transpatellar approach can be done with ease. There is no agreement in whether the plate should be removed after nail placement. It has been our experience that plate retaining does not interfere with early weight-bearing nor time to healing. On the other hand, some biomechanical studies advocate the use of three proximal locking screws instead of two for better construct strength, but with the use of reduction plates (and keeping them in place), just two screws are sufficient to maintain reduction till fracture healing (**Figure 4**) [15].

- Blocking or poller screws: one or more percutaneous blocking screws are positioned after initial insertion of the intramedullary guide. As an easy rule of mind, their position should correspond to where the nail "should not go". 3.5 mm cortical screws or the same screws used for interlocking of the nail can be used. In such manner, during nail insertion, the implant itself can act as a reduction tool, on the condition that a correct starting point has been used. We agree that a nail cannot reduce a proximal tibial fracture by itself. Nonetheless, we think that this can be possible, although only in the setting of proper starting point, trajectory in the proximal fragment, and the use of poller screws (**Figure 5a** and **b**) [14].

When intraarticular extension has occurred in the form of simple split fracture of one or both plateaus, or a simple posterolateral depression fracture, direct or

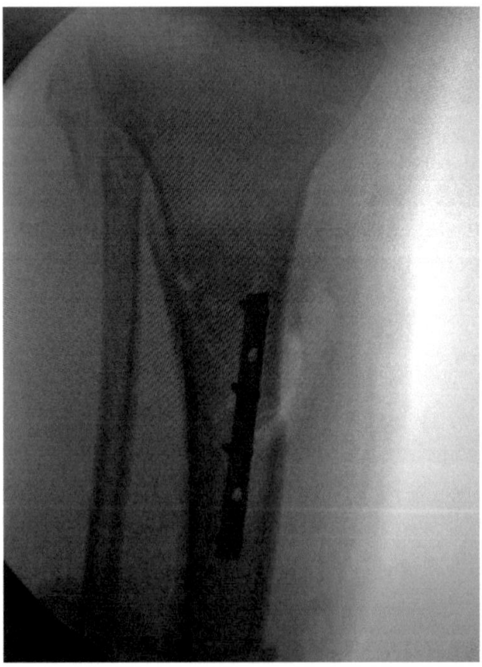

Figure 3.
Direct intraoperative reduction of a proximal comminuted tibial fracture with anterolateral seven-hole 3.5 mm third tubular plate and unicortical screws. This provisional fixation allows maintenance of reduction during reaming and further nail insertion. There is no need for removal of the plate at the completion of the procedure.

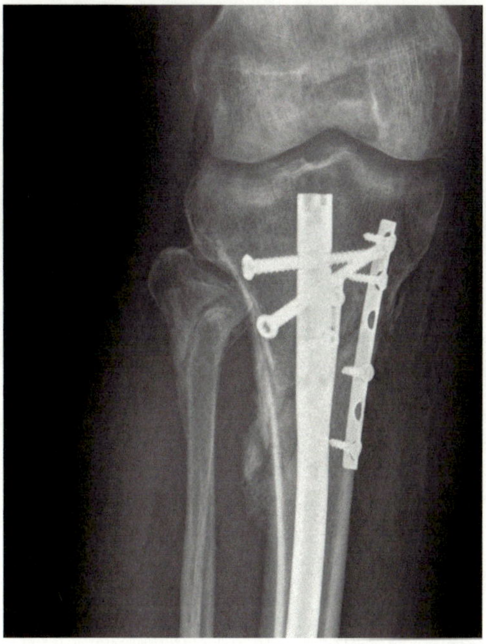

Figure 4.
Proximal tibial fracture in a patient with lupus. Direct reduction and provisional fixation were done with two orthogonal 3.5 mm third tubular plates. Two proximal screws were used for interlocking. Callus and fracture healing maintaining good alignment are seen.

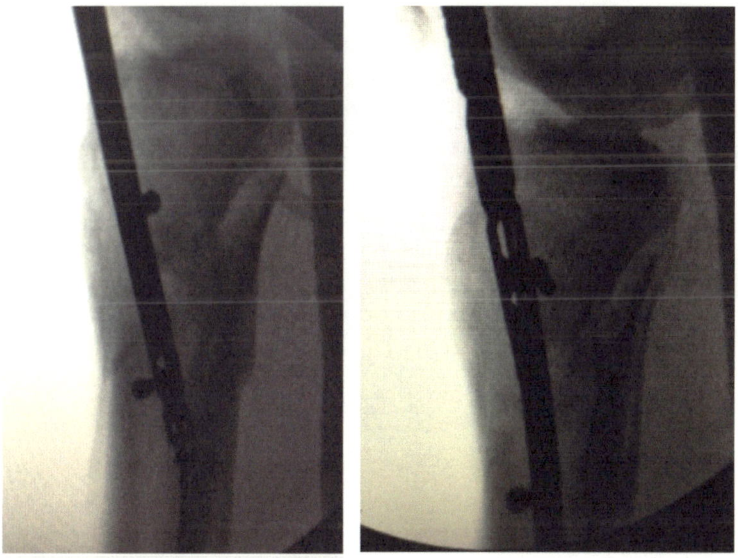

(a) (b)

Figure 5.
(a) The use of poller screws to facilitate reduction in a proximal tibial fracture. After a correct starting point has been made, the position of the two poller screws in this case acts as a lever for the nail to be used as a reduction tool. There is a fulcrum in three points of contact: the two poller screws and the posterior cortex of the distal tibial diaphysis. (b) The three contact points direct the nail distally as – at the same time – it works as a reduction tool. The Herzog angle of the nail has to be taken into account for proper positioning of the poller screws.

indirect reduction and fixation with screws are performed [16]. Positioning of screws should be thoroughly planned, in such a way they do not interfere with the entry point nor trajectory of the nail. This implies that coronal screws should be

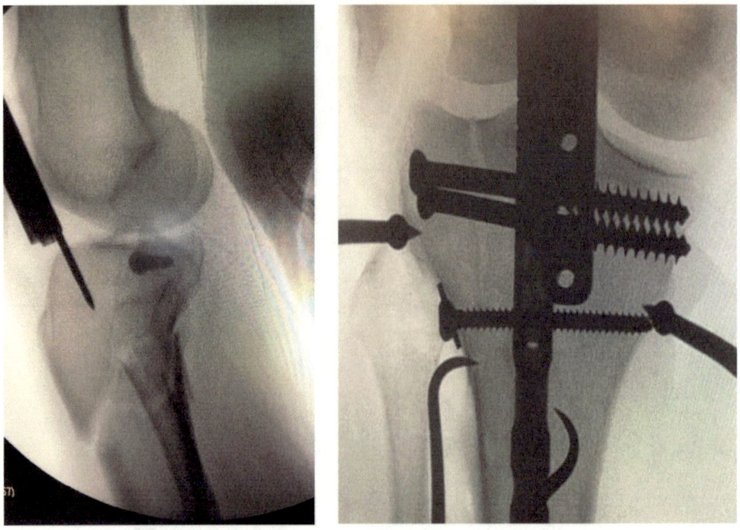

(a) (b)

Figure 6.
(a) A lateral plateau split component of this proximal tibial fracture has been stabilized with a posteriorly placed coronal 6.5 cancellous screw. There is no interference with the entry point of a suprapatellar approach for nail insertion. (b) Suprapatellar nail insertion has been completed. The lateral plateau split was fixed with three large fragment screws. Two percutaneous clamps are in place to help controlling the articular fracture till final interlocking.

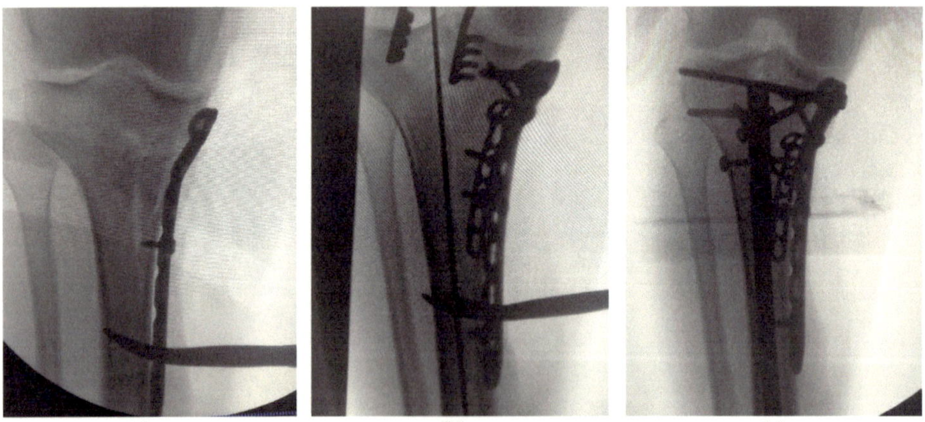

(a) (b) (c)

Figure 7.
(a) Schatzker type VI proximal tibial fracture. Intraoperative management of medial plateau depression and diaphyseal extension with a medial 4.5 mm buttress plate. The unicortical screw secures the plate toward the bone surface, therefore impeding varus deformity at the medial plateau. (b) A second 3.5 mm T-plate was applied as a posteromedial buttress with unicortical screws. Adequate reduction of the proximal tibia is secured in this manner, so a safe conventional transpatellar approach and intramedullary nailing can proceed. (c) After completion of nailing and interlocking, additional fixation of the medial plate is done with screws, engaging the intact lateral plateau.

inserted posteriorly [17]. Transpatellar or suprapatellar approaches are both suitable for this type of injuries (**Figure 6a** and **b**). Articular fractures with diaphyseal extension (Schatzker type VI fractures) might need more complex provisional stabilization in order to maintain continuity between the epiphyseal and diaphyseal components. This can be accomplished with longer unicortical plate applied as buttressing devices (**Figure 7a–c**).

4. Intramedullary nailing of far-distal tibial fractures

Distal meta-epiphyseal tibial fractures account for approximately 15% of distal tibial fractures [18]. As for proximal fractures, plate fixation has been also a well-proven method for treatment. However, the tenuous soft tissue envelope poses a significant limitation for open techniques. As such, percutaneous plating has gained popularity, although more comminuted fractures usually require more than one plate to avoid failure and loss of alignment [19].

Intramedullary nailing, in our appreciation, results in a much solid construct and has shown a very low incidence of failure and loss of angular alignment, due to the location in the center of the axis of the tibia. The most common residual deformity after nailing of the distal tibia is in valgus [20]. We have utilized both supra and transpatellar approach, with similar results in terms of final alignment. Although some authors have reported better alignment indexes when using the suprapatellar approach, others have found that good alignment occurs also with the infrapatellar technique [21]. Various reduction techniques can be used for proper intraoperative reduction: percutaneous reduction clamps [22], limited direct open reduction [23], traction by means of a femoral distractor or by the assistant surgeon, and possibly the use of a suprapatellar approach [13]. In any case, during the procedure, insertion of the intramedullary guide should follow the center of the distal fragment in both anteroposterior and lateral fluoroscopy views [21, 24].

We have distinguished three distinct far-distal fracture patterns to be efficiently managed by locked intramedullary nailing:

a. **Simple oblique or spiral fractures**. In these, a low or intermediate degree of energy causes a fracture line that extends from the metaphyseal area of the distal tibia to the epiphysis but without entering the joint surface of the plafond. At times, more than one fracture line is seen. For preoperative planning, we routinely request a CT scan with 3-D reconstructions [25, 26] (**Figure 8**). This is a valuable tool that allows to depict which might be the location and trajectory of percutaneous screws that maintain the epiphyseal bone block as a whole

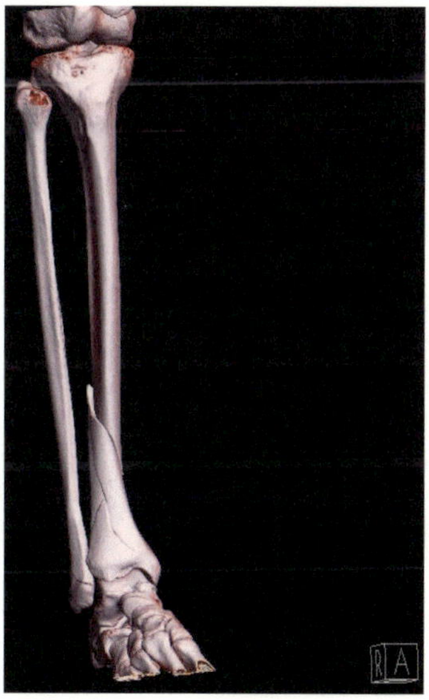

Figure 8.
CT and 3-D reconstruction of a distal tibial fracture with complex spiral epiphyseal extension. The morphology and disposition of the fracture lines can be clearly depicted for proper preoperative planning.

unit, before insertion of the nail. Direct open reduction can be done in selected cases, when anatomical reduction is possible, and the soft tissues are minimally affected by a low-energy fracture pattern [27].

b. **Simple oblique or spiral fractures with articular extension.** These are fractures that include usually a simple split fracture line in the coronal plane or a high medial malleolar fracture, usually both with mild or without displacement. Percutaneous fixation with either 3.5 or 2.7 mm screws prevents articular displacement during final impaction of the nail. At times, the coronal fracture is a split fracture of a large posterior articular fragment in discontinuity with the diaphysis [25, 28]. In these cases, limited open reduction and fixation with a T-shaped 3.5 mm plate are performed, which can be positioned anteriorly or posteriorly prior to nail insertion (**Figure 9a–d**).

c. **Comminuted metaphyseal fractures.** For these, at least two locking screws are needed for stable fixation with a nail. Gorcsyca, in a cadaveric model, showed that two interlocking screws offered similar fixation strength in distal tibial fractures as compared with diaphyseal fractures. In many cases, conventional interlocking screws are enough [24]. Nonetheless, the advent of modern angularly stable locking screws has allowed to improve stability

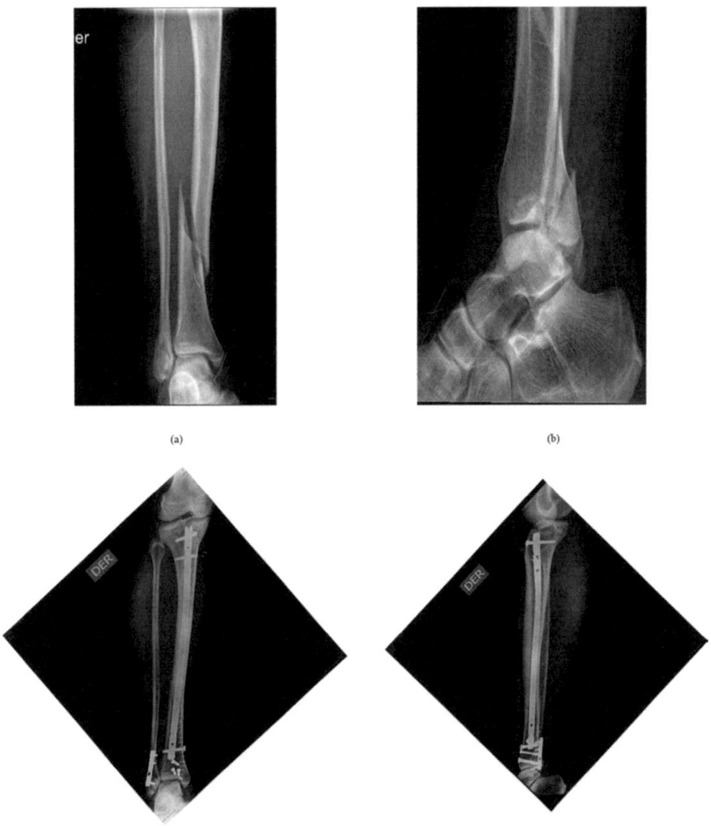

Figure 9.
(a) Anteroposterior radiograph of a distal tibial fracture with a coronal fracture of the posterior malleolus. (b) Lateral view of the lesion, clearly showing the displaced posterior malleolus. (c and d) Anteroposterior and lateral views after direct reduction of the distal fracture with three 4 mm cancellous screws, followed by locked intramedullary nailing and a posterior 3.5 mm third tubular anti-glide plate in the fibula.

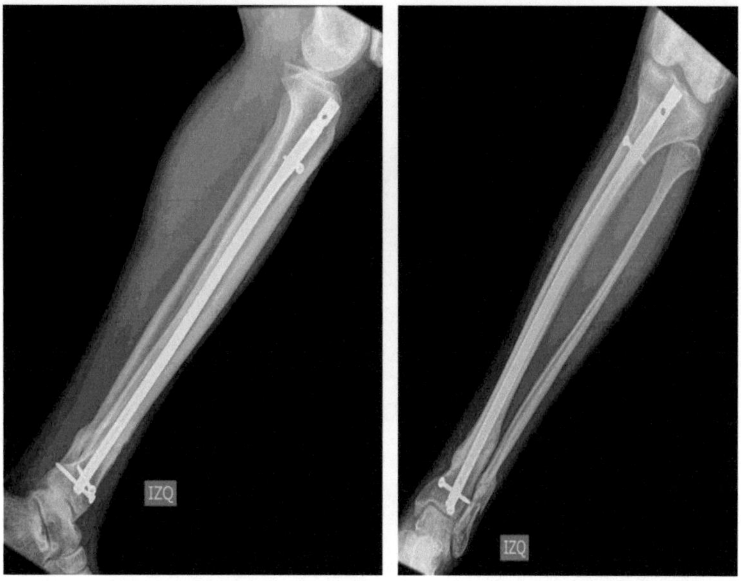

Figure 10.
Follow-up X-rays of a comminuted distal tibial and fibular fracture, treated with nailing and two distal interlocking screws, without fibular fixation. Ankle mortise was stable. Solid tibial fixation alone led to healing without loss of reduction.

even further [29]. Frequently, an associated distal fibular fracture at the same level is present in comminuted distal tibial fractures [28]. Despite that some biomechanical studies have shown that fibular fixation increases the stability of the construct, it is not clear whether this is reflected in better clinical results in long-term follow-up studies [30]. We believe that, if the ankle mortise is not compromised, solid tibial fixation suffices, without the need for osteosynthesis of the fibula (**Figure 10a** and **b**).

5. Fibular fixation in distal tibial fractures

As mentioned before, certain tibial fracture patterns are usually associated with a fractured fibula at the same level. Most of the times, locked intramedullary fixation of the tibia alone is sufficient for proper stability and fracture healing. There is no clear evidence to support the fact that fibular fixation may increase significantly neither the stability of the construct nor the achievement of better clinical outcomes. Moreover, some authors have found that this could increase the rate of nonunion [31]. In a series of 50 patients by Katsenis et al., 31 (62%) had initial fibular fixation with a plate. For the authors, this aided to achieve length, rotation, and alignment of the tibial fracture [32]. We think that there are some fracture patterns that may benefit of fibular fixation, either before or after tibial nailing.

- Comminuted distal tibial fractures and simple fibular fracture: in this case, initial anatomical reduction and fixation of the fibula provide a useful guide for length and rotation of the tibia, which in turn facilitate subsequent tibial nailing (**Figure 11a** and **b**). Care must be taken to correct a tendency for increased varus deformity of the tibial fracture that occurs right after fibular fixation [32].

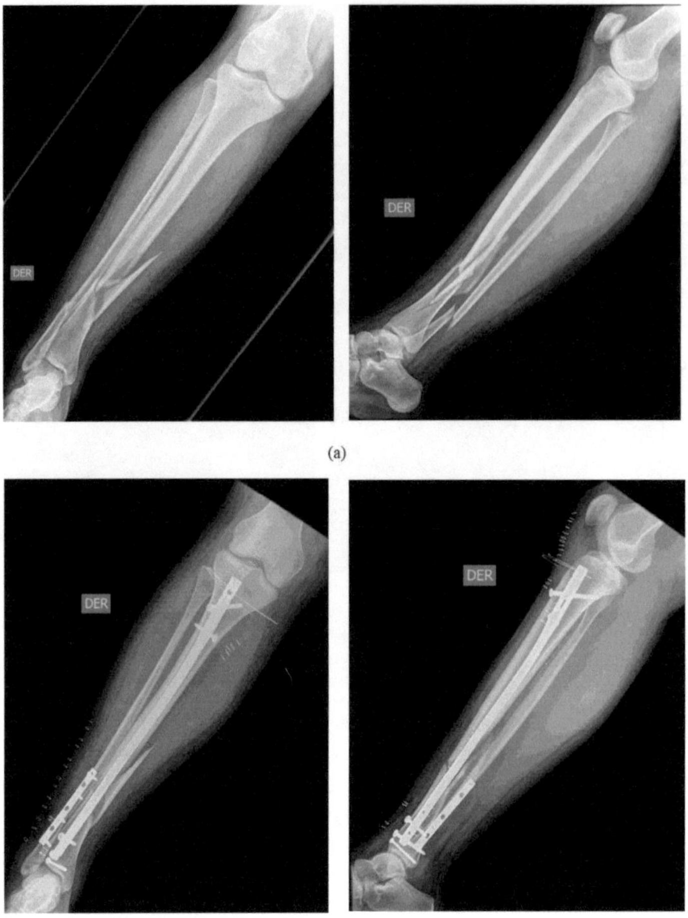

(a)

(b)

Figure 11.
(a) Comminuted distal-fourth open grade I fracture of the right tibia in a 18-year-old female. A simple fibular fracture is seen at the same level. (b) Open reduction and fixation of the fibular fracture with a 3.5 mm third tubular plate were undertaken first, which help with alignment, length, and rotation of the tibia. This was followed by percutaneous fixation of an undisplaced coronal split fracture at the plafond and locked intramedullary tibial nail via transpatellar approach.

- Comminuted distal tibial and fibular fracture at the same level: as aforementioned, despite the fact that intramedullary fixation and distal locking of the tibia suffices, if the surgeon feels that additional fixation of the fibula – and therefore increasing the stability of the construct – might be a benefit (in particular, when distal interlocking of the tibial nail is precarious), this can be carried out easily [33]. For such fixation, we utilize either an axial intramedullary 3.5 mm screw, that is inserted percutaneously, or a 3.5 mm third-tubular plate [30], after tibial fixation is completed. For axial single-screw fixation, we prefer 90 mm or longer, which is available in a pelvic fracture fixation tray. They are both flexible and very stable, providing a secure fibular fixation (**Figure 12a** and **b**).

- Compromise of the ankle mortise: in some cases, tibial fractures at the level of the ankle mortise ligaments result in damage to these restraints and consequent instability. If this event is suspected, after tibial fixation, the stability of the mortise should be tested with stress maneuvers, in order to eventually add fixation and correct this condition (**Figure 13a** and **b**).

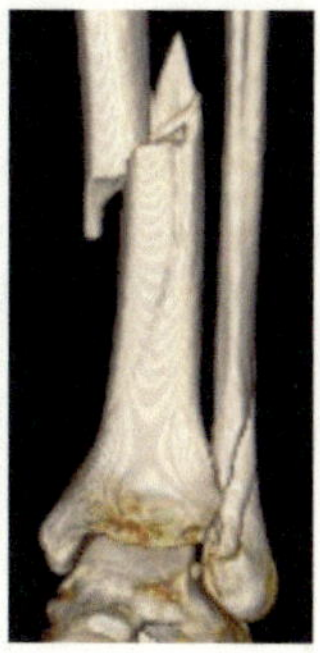

(a)

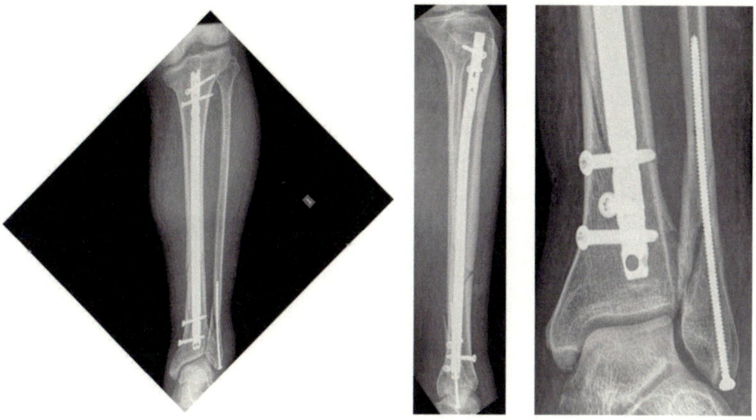

(b)

Figure 12.
(a) A 3-D CT reconstruction of a closed distal tibial fracture with extension toward the metaphysis and a comminuted fibular fracture at the same level. (b) Fixation with locked intramedullary nail and three distal interlocking screws. For additional stability, a percutaneous 3.5 mm long screw was used for fibular fixation.

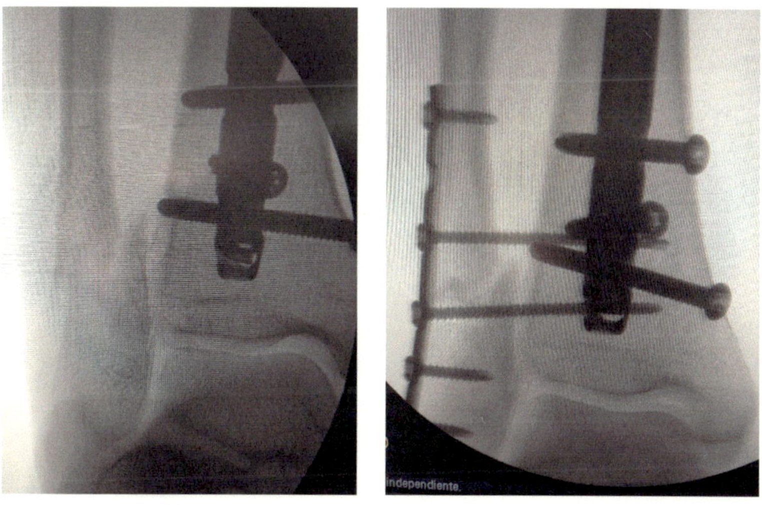

(a) (b)

Figure 13.
(a) In this case, after nail interlocking of a distal tibial fracture, displacement is seen in the distal fibular diaphysis at the level of the mortise, suggesting ankle instability. (b) Fibular fixation with a 3.5 mm third-tubular plate and two syndesmotic screws inserted with compression of the syndesmosis. Appropriate fibular and syndesmosis reduction were obtained.

6. Conclusions

Proximal and distal metaphyseal and meta-epiphyseal tibial fractures have been traditionally managed with either plating techniques – locking or nonlocking – external fixation devices, limited internal fixation in combination with external fixation, and so on.

The indications for locked intramedullary nails have expanded to include these difficult injuries. Essentials for proper fracture alignment and solid fixation are a correct starting point for reaming and nail insertion, maintenance of sound reduction throughout the procedure, and locking screws to secure the nail. Several techniques have been popularized that aid in proper reduction, including the use of blocking or poller screws, limited open direct fracture reduction, and novel surgical approaches for nail insertion, such as the suprapatellar.

The presence of articular extension of fractures, to either one or both tibial plateaus, or the tibial plafond, can be addressed with nails as well. Usually, percutaneous articular reduction and fixation with screws allow to maintain an articular block as a whole and subsequent safe intramedullary fixation.

Clinical outcomes, which are directly related to good anatomical alignment and articular congruency, have been excellent with the use of these methods, giving support for "extreme nailing" techniques for the management of these complex injuries.

Conflict of interest

The authors declare no conflict of interest.

Author details

Luis Bahamonde*, Alvaro Zamorano and Pierluca Zecchetto
Hospital Mutual de Seguridad, University of Chile, Santiago, Chile

*Address all correspondence to: lbahamondemunoz@gmail.com

References

[1] Chand R, Umesh M, Meena K. Intramedullary nailing versus proximal plating in the management of closed extra-articular proximal tibial fracture: A randomized controlled trial. Journal of Orthopaedics and Traumatology. 2015;**16**:203-208

[2] Ryan SP, Steen B, Tornetta P. Semi-extended nailing of metaphyseal tibia fractures: Alignment and incidence of postoperative knee pain. Journal of Orthopaedic Trauma. 2014;**28**(5):263-269

[3] Vallier HA, Le TT, Bedi A. Radiographic and clinical comparisons of distal tibia shaft fractures (4 to 11 cm proximal to the plafond): Plating versus intramedullary nailing. Journal of Orthopaedic Trauma. 2008;**22**(5):307-311

[4] Gopal S, Giannoudis PV, Murray A, Matthews SJ, Smith RM. The functional outcome of severe, open tibial fractures managed with early fixation and flap coverage. Journal of Bone and Joint Surgery. 2004;**86**:861-867

[5] Redfern DJ, Syed SU, Davies SJM. Fractures of the distal tibia: Minimally invasive plate osteosynthesis. Injury. 2004;**35**:615-620

[6] Virkus WW, Kempton LB, Sorkin AT, Gaski GE. Intramedullary nailing of periarticular fractures. Journal of the American Academy of Orthopaedic Surgeons. 2018;**26**(18):629-639

[7] Hak DJ. Intramedullary nailing of proximal third tibial fractures: Techniques to improve reduction. Orthopedics. 2011;**34**(7):532-535

[8] Liporace FA, Stadler CM, Yoon RS. Problems, tricks, and pearls in intramedullary nailing of proximal third tibial fractures. Journal of Orthopaedic Trauma. 2013;**27**(1):56-62

[9] Zelle BA, Boni G. Safe surgical technique: Intramedullary nail fixation of tibial shaft fractures. Patient Safety in Surgery. 2015;**9**:40

[10] Stinner DJ, Mir H. Techniques for intramedullary nailing of proximal tibia fractures. Orthopedic Clinics of North America. 2014;**45**(1):33-45. DOI: 10.1016/j.ocl.2013.09.001

[11] Chen X, Xu H, Zhang H, Chen J. Suprapatellar versus infrapatellar intramedullary nailing for treatment of tibial shaft fractures in adults. Medicine. 2018;**97**(32):e11799

[12] Jia P, Lu F, Ullah K, Zhang M, Dong Y, Xiong C. Angle stable interlocking intramedullary nails for tibial plateau fractures. Orthopaedic Surgery. 2018;**10**(2):115-120

[13] Brink O. Suprapatellar nailing of tibial fractures: Surgical hints. Current Orthopaedic Practice. 2016;**27**(1):107-112

[14] Ricci WM, Boyle MO, Borrelli J, Bellabarba C, Sanders R. Fractures of the proximal third of the tibial shaft treated with intramedullary nails and blocking screws. Journal of Orthopaedic Trauma. 2001;**15**(4):264-270

[15] Hiesterman D. Intramedullary nailing of extra- articular proximal tibia fractures. Journal of the American Academy of Orthopaedic Surgeons. 2011;**19**:690-700

[16] Högel F, Hoffmann S, Panzer S, Wimber JBV. Biomechanical comparison of intramedullar versus extramedullar stabilization of intra-articular tibial plateau fractures. Archives of Orthopaedic and Trauma Surgery. 2013;**133**:59-64

[17] Kubiak EN, Camuso MR, Barei DP, Frcs C, Nork SE. Operative

treatment of ipsilateral noncontiguous unicondylar tibial plateau and shaft fractures: Combining plates and nails. Journal of Orthopaedic Trauma. 2008;**22**(C):560-565

[18] Wennergren AD, Bergdahl C, Ekelund J, Juto H, Sundfeldt M, Michael M. Epidemiology and incidence of tibia fractures in the Swedish fracture register. Injury. 2018;**49**(11):2068-2074. DOI: 10.1016/j.injury.2018.09.008

[19] Hu L, Xiong Y, Mi B, Panayi AC, Zhou W, Liu Y, et al. Comparison of intramedullary nailing and plate fixation in distal tibial fractures with metaphyseal damage: A meta-analysis of randomized controlled trials. Journal of Orthopaedic Surgery and Research. 2019;**1**:1-11

[20] Newman SDS, Mauffrey CPC, Krikler S. Distal metadiaphyseal tibial fractures. Injury. 2011;**42**:975-984

[21] Richard RD, Kubiak E, Horwitz DS. Techniques for the surgical treatment of distal tibia fractures distal tibia fractures surgical treatment open reduction internal fixation. Orthopedic Clinics of North America. 2014;**45**(3):295-312. DOI: 10.1016/j.ocl.2014.04.001

[22] Cory A, Collinge MD, Michael J, Beltran MD, Henry A, Dollahite BS, et al. Percutaneous clamping of spiral and oblique fractures of the tibial shaft: A safe and effective reduction aid during intramedullary nailing. Journal of Orthopaedic Trauma. 2015;**29**(6):e208-e212

[23] Auston DA, Meiss J, Serrano R, Sellers T, Carlson G, Hoggard T, et al. Percutaneous or open reduction of closed tibial shaft fractures during intramedullary nailing does not increase wound complications , infection or nonunion rates. Journal of Orthopaedic Trauma. 2017;**31**(4):215-219

[24] Rommens PM, Küchle R, Hofmann A. MHH. Intramedullary nailing of metaphyseal fractures of the lower extremity. Acta Chirurgiae Orthopaedicae et Traumatologiae Cechoslovaca. 2017;**84**(5):330-340

[25] Zhang Y, Qin X, Song L, Li X. The risk of violating the posterior malleolar fracture when nailing the ipsilateral concomitant spiral distal tibial fracture. BMC Musculoskeletal Disorders. 2018;**19**:123

[26] Purnell GJ, Glass ER, Altman DT, Sciulli RL, Muffly MT, Altman GT. Results of a computed tomography protocol evaluating distal third tibial shaft fractures to assess noncontiguous malleolar fractures. Journal of Trauma, Injury, Infection, and Critical Care. 2011;**71**(1):163-168

[27] Gupta RK, Rohilla RK. Locking plate fixation in distal metaphyseal tibial fractures: Series of 79 patients. International Orthopaedics. 2010;**34**:1285-1290

[28] Robinson CM, Mclauchlan GJ, Mclean IP. Distal metaphyseal fractures of the tibia with minimal involvement of the ankle. Journal of Bone and Joint Surgery. 1995;**77**(5):781-787

[29] Wähnert D, Stolarczyk Y, Hofmann GO, Mückley T. The primary stability of angle-stable versus conventional locked intramedullary nails. International Orthopaedics. 2012;**36**:1059-1064

[30] Varsalona R. Distal tibial metaphyseal fractures: The role of fibular fixation. Strategies in Trauma and Limb Reconstruction. 2006;**1**:42-50

[31] Berlusconi M, Busnelli L, Chiodini F, Portinaro N. To fix or not to fix? The role of fibular fixation in distal shaft fractures of the leg. Injury. 2014;**45**(2):408-411. DOI: 10.1016/j.injury.2013.09.017

[32] Katsenis DL, Begkas D, Spiliopoulos G, Stamoulis D. The results of closed intramedullary nailing for intra-articular distal tibial fractures. Journal of Orthopaedic Trauma. 2014;**28**(2):108-113

[33] Khan R, Jameel J, Kumar S, Aslam A, Chahal G, Rastogi S. Rush nail in the management of distal one-third fibular fracture in both bone fractured legs: A clinical study. Journal of Bone and Join Diseases. 2017;**32**(2):32-36

Section 3

Suggestions for Therapy (Conservative or Surgical) before Joint Arthroplasty

Chapter 5

The Regenerative Effect of Intra-Articular Injection of Autologous Fat Micro-Graft in Treatment of Chronic Knee Osteoarthritis

Sabah S. Moshref, Yasir S. Jamal, Amro M. Al-Hibshi and Abdullah M. Kaki

Abstract

The study started in 2010 to find the effect of autologous fat micrograft for osteoarthritis (OA); the result was published on normal animal's model, in 10 patients, then in 80 patients with knee osteoarthritis, and the current study in 205 patients. The study was conducted at King Abdulaziz University Hospital (January 2012–October 2015); 80 adult patients were suffering from moderate to severe knee osteoarthritis. About 10–20 mL fat micrograft was prepared with liposuction and injected intra-articularly into the affected knee/s. The results revealed that pain improvement after the fat injection during rest and with activity with the visual analogue scale. The Western Ontario and McMaster Universities Osteoarthritis Index (WOMAC) indicated improvement, both in the three domains (pain, stiffness, and physical function) and in total. The use of intra-articular autologous fat micrograft is simple, safe, and effective for degenerative knee osteoarthritis.

Keywords: autologous fat micrograft, intra-articular injection, knee osteoarthritis, cartilage degeneration, regenerative therapy repair

1. Introduction

Fat grafting and its use in aesthetic and reconstructive surgeries are considered a state of art, but looking back at the history, it is just a revival in the techniques, which was described previously by others when **Gustav Neuber** on 1893 was the first to perform fat graft for orbital depression in human and Erich Lexer who is a skilled German orthopedic and plastic surgeon reported a variety of clinical uses of fat graft in management of knee ankylosis and fat graft wrapped around the tendon during tendon repair to prevent skin tendon adhesion and restore gliding [1, 2].

The revolution in surgical specialty directed toward minimally invasive therapeutic modalities where endoscopic surgery replaced the open surgical operations; similarly, the recent discovery of the regenerative effect of fat micrograft due to presence of adipose-derived stem cells (ADSCs), cytokines, growth factors, pre adipocytes, and mature adipocytes led to a growing interest for the use fat graft as regenerative treatment replacing the major surgical rejuvenative operation, and Liu et al. [3] in his major review article, which includes over 265 clinical trials about therapeutic application of mesenchymal stem cells (MSCs) for common bone and joint diseases, indicated that the MSCs are considered as an ideal source of cell therapy for different types of diseases including bone and joint diseases [3–5].

In this chapter we present our experience over the current decade in management of osteoarthritis (OA) by intra-articular injection of fat micrograft (IAFMG), describing our approach, which was developed from the belief in the powerful reparative effect of autologous fat graft for damage tissue as well as natural lubricating effect on the joints. We started on animal model, and upon confirming its safety and positive regenerative effects, we applied this minimally invasive modality on patients with advanced and moderate chronic osteoarthritis with fulfillment of ethical approval requirement for the trials on human subjects. The satisfactory outcome of this minimally invasive modality indicates that intra-articular injection of fat micrograft can replace or delay considerably the need for the classical major joint replacement surgery (JRS), with its impact on the quality of life of patients and financial cost of JRS, and long hospitalization and absence of work when compared to our minimally invasive procedure [6, 7].

2. Disease characteristics

Chronic osteoarthritis is a common complex disorder affecting middle-aged and elderly females more than males but all races. The main risk factors are constitutional, including sedentary lifestyle, obesity and aging, and genetic and local factors (biomechanical consequences of joint injury, joint laxity, or malalignment). Therefore, the stress from mechanical force plays an important critical role in the initiation and progression of the disease; it is also associated with chronic disease such as diabetes, gout, and poor diet [8–15].

Osteoarthritis is the disease of the whole joint, including the bone, cartilage, tendons, ligaments, synovium, and synovial fluid. Osteoarthritis mainly affects weight-bearing joints (i.e., knees, hips, or spine) due to chronic high stress, which leads to degradation of the cartilage; subchondral cysts; sclerosis, which stimulates new bone outgrowths (osteophytes); and synovitis leading to reduction of joint viscosity and lubrication with more friction, irritation, consequently more cartilage damage and effusion, ligament laxity and meniscal tears, and progressive narrowing of joint space. The usual patient presentation is joint pain, swelling, crepitus, morning joint stiffness, and, after prolonged rest, hyperthermia, progressively restricted movement, and major disability with deterioration in quality of life [9, 10, 16, 17].

3. Management

Management included the diagnosis of the disease and its extent based on clinical presenting symptoms and signs of the patient, evaluating the degree of pain, mobility, and functions of the diseased joint, and then utilizing the radiological modalities to confirm the disease and its severity with plain X-ray, CT scan, MRI, and other available imaging modalities; following clinical and radiological diagnoses, the plan of treatment is established according to the extent of the disease, which is ranging from nonsurgical to minimally invasive or major surgical procedure.

4. Nonsurgical therapy

Currently there is no curative intervention; all treatment modalities are directed toward pain control, improvement of joint mobility and functions, and avoiding drugs with adverse effects. Non-pharmacological management should include a combination approach in the form of patient education, modification of lifestyle, self-management, weight reduction, exercise, conventional physiotherapy, electrotherapy, hydrotherapy, and occupational therapy to prevent excessive stress on the joint.

The pharmacological symptomatic therapies for pain control are in the form of nonsteroidal anti-inflammatory medications such as acetaminophen and COX-2-specific inhibitors and topical nonsteroidal anti-inflammatory drugs. On the other hand, intra-articular injection of corticosteroids and viscous supplementation injections of hyaluronic acid improve pain and viscosity, but these pharmacological treatments have short-term improvement effect and are costly, and the intra-articular injections have a risk of acute synovitis [18–23].

Recently, the intra-articular injection of platelet-rich plasma to human osteo-arthritic joints associated with significant clinical symptomatic improvements of inflammation and pain and viscosity [24].

5. Surgical therapy

Surgical therapy included minor and major surgical operations, but the recent use of the minimally invasive surgical procedure of intra-articular injection fat micro-graft with the contained adipose-derived stem cells, which we studied on animal model followed by human joints, showed very satisfactory outcome; this modality of treatment is the main theme of this chapter which will be discussed in details.

The minor surgical procedures include arthroscopic joint lavage debridement, which demonstrated short-term symptom relief with more improvement when combined with marrow-stimulating microfracture and drilling procedures of articular surface; this improvement in joint functions would postpone the need for knee replacement [25].

6. The major surgical procedures

On the other hand, joint replacement as major surgical intervention is reserved for patients with failure of other modalities and in patients with joint end-stage disease, as joint implants have a finite life span (~10–15 years). After that a variety of complications might occur such as wear particle formation, which contribute to loosening which required revision surgery; therefore the use of artificial joints in young patients (e.g., <55 years) is associated with higher revision rates of this operation with its associated disadvantages as being a major procedure with complications, long hospitalization, absence from work, and high cost, which indicate the need to develop new treatment options. Therefore tissue engineering regeneration offers a long-term solution for repair of the affected tissue components of the joints such as the bone, ligament, and knee meniscus [26–28].

7. The stem cell line therapy

Osteoarthritis is an active disease process with an imbalance between the repair and destruction and degeneration of joint with poor intrinsic healing power and regeneration due to poor vascularization and absence of direct access to progenitor cells of bone marrow [29].

For many years, researchers have been seeking to understand the body's ability to repair and replace the damaged tissues; these researches led them to the discovery of the unique mesenchymal stem cell, which is partly responsible for maintenance and repairing of damaged connective tissues after injury. They can migrate toward injured tissues, where they display trophic effects of synthesis of proliferative, proangiogenic, and regenerative molecules. Mesenchymal stem cells undergo site-specific differentiation into a variety of connective tissues including cartilage, bone, fat, tendon, ligament, marrow stroma, and others, with its reparative and regenerative effects with anti-inflammatory and immunomodulatory actions via direct cell-cell interaction or secretion of bioactive factors, resulting in differentiation, stemness maintenance, self-renewal, prevention, and modification of progress of the disease [17, 30–38].

Mesenchymal stem cells can be isolated from several human sources other than the bone marrow and fetal tissues, including adipose tissue (ADSCs) with similar phenotypic characteristics but different propensities in proliferation and differentiation potentials, and provide an abundant and easily accessible source of stem cells [39–46].

With all these properties, MSCs are considered as an ideal source of cell therapy for different types of diseases including bone and joint diseases as reviewed by Liu et al. [3] as a review article about therapeutic application of MSCs for common bone and joint diseases, which include over 265 clinical trials of MSCs registered with clinical trial for knee osteoarthritis and other joint and bone diseases; they conclude that MSC is a promising prospect in clinical application for bone and joint diseases, without any reports of post application adverse immune side effects [5].

8. Animal and human researches on uses of MSCs in joints

With the growing interest of using MSCs as biological treatment for cartilage repair in arthritic joint diseases on different animal models where stem cells grown on different media scaffolds include synthetic or natural extracellular matrix, implantation of stem cells into the joints is either as invasive via arthroscopy with possible increased risk of infection or noninvasive intra-articular injection MSCs. These trials are summarized in **Table 1** [6, 46–59].

Animal model trial				
Publication	**MSCs**	**Description**	**Intervention**	**Outcome**
Murphy et al. [46]	BMC	MSC and suspension of hyaluronan injected in goat OA joint Intra-articular injection	Minimally invasive	+ Cartilage regeneration
Guo et al. [47]	BMC	MSCs grow on scaffolds of bioceramic beta-tricalcium phosphate via open arthrotomy	Invasive with risk of infection	Marked improvement
Hui et al. [48]	BMC	MSCs grow on scaffolds of fibrin glue by open arthrotomy implantation	Invasive with risk of infection	Marked improvement
Liu et al. [49]	BMC	MSCs grow on scaffolds of hyaluronic acid and gelatin by open arthrotomy	Invasive risk of infection	Marked improvement

Animal model trial				
Publication	**MSCs**	**Description**	**Intervention**	**Outcome**
Kayakabe et al. [50]	BMC	MSCs grow on scaffold of hyaluronic gel sponge by open arthrotomy	Invasive with risk of infection	Marked improvement
Yan et al. [51]	BMC	MSCs grow on scaffolds of polylactic acid by open arthrotomy	Invasive with risk of infection	Marked improvement
Lee et al. [52]	BMC	MSC and suspension of hyaluronan in injected mini pig OA joint Intra-articular injection	Minimally invasive	+Cartilage regeneration
Kuroda et al. [53]	BMC	MSCs grow on scaffolds of collagen gel by open arthrotomy	Invasive with risk of infection	+Cartilage regeneration
Black et al. [54, 55]	ADMSCs	Double-blinded, placebo-controlled clinical trial on the effect? IN dogs with chronic OA of the coxofemoral and humeroradial joints Intra-articular injection	Minimally invasive	Significant improvement
Noth et al. [56]	BMC	MSCs seeded on three-dimensional biodegradable scaffolds Intra-articular injection	Minimally invasive	+Cartilage regeneration
Horie et al. [57]	Synovium MSCs	Synovium MSCs in massive meniscal defect knee rat intra-articular injection	Minimally invasive	Promoted meniscal regeneration
Mokbel et al. [58]	BMC	MSC and suspension of hyaluronan in donkey Intra-articular injection	Minimally invasive	+Cartilage regeneration
Sato et al. [59]	BMC	MSC and suspension of hyaluronan in Hartley strain guinea pig Intra-articular injection	Minimally invasive	+Cartilage regeneration
Moshref et al. [6]	ADMSCs	Intra-articular injection of autologous fat micrograft **in normal** sheep hind joints, intra-articular injection	Minimally invasive	Increase of the articular hyaline cartilage thickness Significant chondrocyte proliferation

Table 1.
The other animal model trial studies.

9. Our animal trial

Our study started as an idea on 2010, when we plan to use autologous fat micrograft for treatment of osteoarthritis and we started by injecting fat micrograft into normal hind joints of sheep to determine the safety and effects of intra-articular injection of autologous fat micrograft, followed by observing the animal's activities in using their injected joints, and by examining any macroscopic or microscopic changes in the articular cartilage of the fat-injected joints compared to other similar

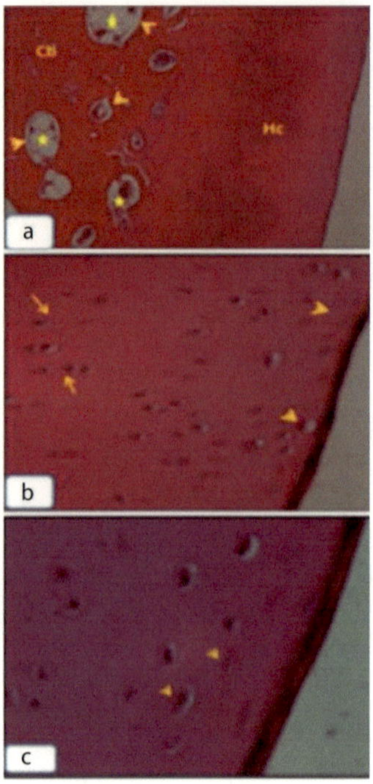

Figure 1.
(a–c) The control sheep H&E stain; longitudinal sections in femoral diarthrosis of left hind knee. (a) Normal histological structure of the articular hyaline cartilage (Hc) compact bone (Cb), spongy bone (head arrows), and bone marrow (*), 100×. (b, c) Flattened chondrocytes (head arrows) of the surface layer of hyaline cartilage followed by internal globular chondrocytes arranged in rows (arrows), 400×; 1000×.

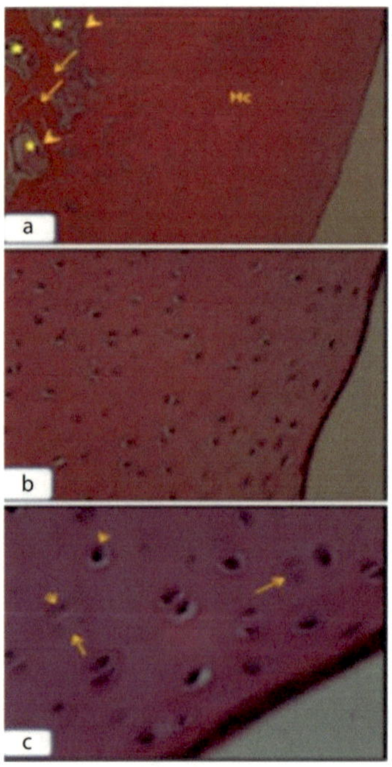

Figure 2.
(a–c) The treated sheep right hind knee; longitudinal sections in femoral diarthrosis H&E stain. (a) Increasing the thickness of the articular hyaline cartilage (Hc) layer; compact bone (arrows), spongy bone (head arrows), and bone marrow (*) were observed in normal view, 100×. (b) Increasing the number of chondrocytes (arrows), 400×. (c) Chondrocyte division, metaphase (head arrows), telophase (arrows) 1000×.

Knee Joints	Femoral diarthrosis	Tibial diarthrosis
Control	40.90 ± 0.432 Left joints	42.72 ± 0.700
Treated	55.31 ± 0.681[**] Right joint	49.10 ± 0.585[*]

[*]*Significant at* $p \leq 0.01$.
[**]*High significant at* $p \leq 0.001$.

Table 2.
Number of chondrocytes in control and treated articular cartilage of sheep knee joints.

non-injected joint of the same animal; the study confirmed the safety, without any associated detrimental effects, on the joint tissues. Furthermore, it had positive microscopic findings as there was increase of the thickness of the articular hyaline cartilage layer with significant proliferation of chondrocytes including different mitosis stages (**Figures 1** and **2**, **Table 2**). Therefore, intra-articular injection of fat micrograft is an ideal minimally invasive choice for joint lubrication with high potential healing effects.

10. Our human trial

After the successful encouraging results of our previous animal study, which demonstrates the potential healing power and regenerative effect of autologous fat micrograft with its stem cells and all other study reports of clinical trials and publication by using mesenchymal stromal/stem cells for management of osteoarthritis, which offer a great hope for the treatment of osteoarthritic joints, we decided to evaluate the efficacy of fresh non-processed autologous fat micrograft with its ADSCs for management of osteoarthritic joints as prospective interventional clinical trial, which was conducted at King Abdulaziz University Hospital, Jeddah, Saudi Arabia, after obtaining the ethical approval from the local research and ethics committee, No. 822-12, according to latest vision of the Declaration of Helsinki. Over the period of 2012–2013, a preliminary clinical trial was conducted on 10 adult patients of both genders suffering from severe to moderate knee osteoarthritis with encouraging results as an effective and safe method for the treatment of knee osteoarthritis, then we expand the trial on 80 adult patients which confirm our previous finding, and then the clinical trial concluded with the final reporting to ethical committee on December 2016 [2, 3, 6, 7, 66].

But our work in utilizing this modality of treatment continued, and we are currently presenting the outcome in 205 adult patients (392 knee joints) who were managed and completed the required period of follow-up [7, 60–75, 77, 78].

The other studies were mainly revolving around the use of bone marrow or expanded adipose tissues and non-expanded autologous MSCs although some trials use allogenic MSCs. Most researchers focus on the use of intra-articular injections without the use of scaffolds or major surgeries since injections are more cost-effective, have little morbidity, and are a desirable way of treatment. The satisfactory outcome of our study over 10 years indicated that MSC treatment appears to be a good option for treatment of moderate to severe OA in the elderly; other studies reported similar results to ours in demonstrating promising prospect of cell therapy in many refractory diseases, including bone and joint diseases, in great improvement of pain, mobility, and other joint functions; these have high potential for clinical use in tissue engineering and regenerative and reparative medicine. Other studies found MSCs effective in cartilage healing; these trials are summarized in **Table 3** [28, 70–73, 76].

Human clinical studies				
Publication	**Type of MSCs**	**Description**	**Intervention**	**Outcome**
Davatchi et al. [76]	BMC	MSCs injected with autologous BMSCs intra-articularly of four patients	Minimally invasive	Marked improvement
Wakitani et al. [70]	BMC Human autologous culture expanded	MSC embedded in collagen gel injected into medial femoral condyle of 12 patients and 12 as control	Invasive with risk of infection	Marked improvement
Ohgushi et al. [71]	BMC	MSC seeded at ceramic ankle prosthesis and injected in the three-severe arthritic ankle for patients	Invasive with risk of infection	Marked improvement
Centeno et al. [72]	BMC	MSCs injected intra-articularly for 46-A case report study year	Minimally invasive	Marked improvement
Buda et al. [73]	BMC Human autologous culture expanded	MSC and hyaluronic acid for 20 patients (12 males and eight females)	Minimally invasive	Marked improvement
Pak et al. [74, 75]	ADSCs	MSC and hyaluronic acid, calcium chloride, a nanogram dose of dexamethasone, and platelet-rich plasma injected intra-articularly for knee osteoarthritis or hip osteonecrosis	Minimally invasive	Marked clinical improvement and cartilage thickening
Koh et al. [77]	ADSCs Infrapatellar fat pad	Autologous AMSCs from infrapatellar fat pad injected at intra-articular injection for 25 patients	Minimally invasive	Significant regeneration of cartilage
Koh et al. [78]	ADSCs Infrapatellar fat pad	AMSCs autologous injection intra-articular of 18 patients	Minimally invasive	Marked improvement
Moshref et al. [7]	ADSCs	Intra-articular injection of autologous fat micrograft for the treatment of knee osteoarthritis Preliminary trail of 10 patients	Minimally invasive	Significant clinical improvement
Moshref et al. [66]	ADSCs	Intra-articular injection of autologous fat micrograft for the treatment of knee osteoarthritis. 80 patients and 148 joints	Minimally invasive	Significant clinical improvement
Moshref 2019 (under consideration)	ADSCs	Intra-articular injection of autologous fat micrograft for the treatment of knee osteoarthritis. 205 patients and 392 joints	Minimally invasive	Significant clinical improvement

Table 3.
The other human clinical studies.

11. Study guidelines and patient selection

- **Patients**: all patients were adult patients from both genders and were screened for eligibility to participate in the study; each patient underwent a complete medical history, a physical examination, and a full assessment of the joint.

- **Informed written consent** was obtained from each patient before treatment after explaining to him all about the study and this modality of treatment.
- **Inclusion criteria**: all cases of severe to moderate knee osteoarthritis, the changes to be confirmed by bilateral anterior-posterior standing and lateral supine radiographs involving one or both knees.
- **Exclusion criteria**: recent knee surgery, chronic opioid intake, bleeding disorders, malignant disease, congenital or traumatic deformity of the knee joint, and refusal of the patient to be included in the study.
- **For the evaluation of patient**, we used **the visual analogue scale** for pain assessment (on scale 0–10 cm line, 0 = no pain and 10 = worst imaginable pain) was explained to patients during the preoperative visit; visual analogue scale at rest and during activity was obtained.
- **The Western Ontario and McMaster Universities Osteoarthritis Index** (WOMAC) is a questionnaire widely used to assess the symptoms and physical disability associated with osteoarthritis; we used five-point Likert-type Western Ontario and McMaster Universities Osteoarthritis Index to collect information regarding the three subscales of Western Ontario and McMaster Universities Osteoarthritis Index. Pain (five items): while sitting or lying, walking, using stairs, standing, and in bed. Stiffness (two items): after first walking and later in the day. Physical function (17 items): standing, walking, sitting, rising from sitting, stair use, bending, putting on or taking off socks, lying in bed, rising from bed, getting in or out of the bath, sitting on or rising from the toilet, getting in or out of a car, shopping, light household duties, and heavy household duties
- **Anesthesia and surgical interventions** were explained to the patients. A list of adverse effects was reviewed with the patients to allow for reporting of any side effect that may arise post-procedure.

12. Anesthesia

The procedures were performed under controlled local anesthesia and sedation. Dexmedetomidine 0.7 mcg/kg/hour was administered intravenously as a sedative and pain reliever. Patients were monitored for heart rate, pulse oximetry, temperature, and noninvasive blood pressure.

13. Procedures

The surgical site of liposuction was carefully chosen based on the availability of fat and the patients' wishes. Liposuction was performed under complete aseptic technique and antibiotic coverage of cefuroxime 1.5 g IV one dose, 1 hour preoperative followed by 500 mg orally every 12 hours for 7 days. Fat harvesting was obtained using 10-hole, Olivaire blunt cannula (Pouret Medical, Clichy, France) with 1 mm tip attached to a 10 mL Luer-Lok syringe (Terumo, Auburn, WA, USA). Fifty milliliters of fat micrograft was collected and then left for thirty minutes to settle and separate into various layers; the upper and lower layers were removed, while the middle layer of fat was kept for intra-articular injection (**Figure 1**).

The surgical site was prepared and injected with 100–200 mL of tumescent solution. Solution was prepared by mixing 30–50 mL of 1% lidocaine and 0.5 mg (0.5 mL) of epinephrine in 449.5 mL of lactated ringers. The osteoarthritic knee joint was injected with autologous intra-articular fat micrograft 15–20 mL through the lateral approach according to the case in an amount that did not produce high pressure inside the joint and did not produce pain to the patients due to tension of the joint capsule.

14. Postoperative advice and care

- After operation, the patient received antibiotics at home for 1 week and on regular pain killer for 2 weeks and is to start walking immediately as early as possible and increase activity as tolerated.

- Stress the preoperative advice to reduce weight, improve diet regimen, and perform regular exercise especially aqua or hydrotherapy therapy to strengthen muscle with consequently more improvement of outcome of the procedure.

- All patients were followed up in the clinic on a regular basis every 1–2 weeks in the first month and then every 3 months to assess incidence of side effects, complications, pain evaluation, stiffness and knee function problems, and recurrence of pain.

- The patient was informed that the improvement will start during the first month and increase with time, and the maximum appreciated improvement at 6 months, provided he will follow the given instructions and improve the predisposing risk and comorbid factors.

15. Statistical analysis

IBM SPSS Statistics for Windows, Version 20 (IBM Corp., Armonk, NY USA), was used for data analysis. Data were presented as mean ± SD and minimum-maximum or number and percentage (n, %) as appropriate. Wilcoxon test for nonparametric variables was used to compare preinjection to postinjection values. A probability of ≤ 0.05 was considered significant.

16. The current study outcome of 205 patients

In this current study, we used the same methodology and patient's selection that we applied in the preliminary trial and in the main study of 80 patients indicated in the requested ethical approval, but in this chapter, we are presenting our experience in the management of 205 patients.

Table 4 showed the demographic data and the clinical characteristics of the patients. The median age of the patients was 61.59 years, and the body mass index was 35.10 kg/m^2. The female patients were more than male (74.10% versus 25.90%) with a ratio of 2.88:1. Only five patients (2.90%) were smoking. The associated comorbidities were obesity (74.60%), hypertension (34.60%), *diabetes mellitus* (21.50%), hypothyroidism (6.80%), rheumatoid arthritis (4.90%), low back pain (4.90%), hepatitis (2.00%), and lower limb edema (1.50%).

Parameters	Data
Age (years)	61.59 ± 10.32 (33–92)
Weight (kg)	87.25 ± 16.89 (48–164)
Height (meter)	1.56 ± 0.10 (1.14–1.86)
Body mass index (kg/m^2)	35.10 ± 5.77 (22.00–50.60)
Gender	
Male	53 (25.90%)
Female	152 (74.10%)
Smoking	5 (2.90%)
Comorbidity	
Obesity	153 (74.60%)
Hypertension	71 (34.60%)
Type 2 *diabetes mellitus*	44 (21.50%)
Hypothyroidism	14 (6.80%)
Rheumatoid arthritis	10 (4.90%)
Low back pain	10 (4.90%)
Lower limb edema	3 (1.50%)
Hepatitis	4 (2.00%)

Data are expressed as mean ± SD (minimum-maximum) or number (%) as appropriate.

Table 4.
Demographic and clinical characteristics of patients (n = 205).

Parameters	Data
Disease duration (years)	8.00 ± 5.98 (1.00–33.00)
Knee affected	
Right knee	13 (6.30%)
Left knee	5 (2.40%)
Bilateral knees	187 (91.20%)
Medications	
Nonsteroidal anti-inflammatory	204 (99.50%)
Glucosamine	18 (8.80%)
Prednisone	10 (4.90%)
Methotrexate	7 (3.40%)
Relaxon	9 (4.40%)
Fat injection	
Single injection	199 (97.10%)
Two injections	5 (2.40%)
Three injections	1 (0.50%)

Data are expressed as mean ± SD (minimum-maximum) or number (%) as appropriate.

Table 5.
Disease duration and treatment of patients (n = 205).

The duration of OA ranged from 1 to 33 years. The right knee was affected in 6.30% of patients and left knee in 2.40%, while both knees were affected in 91.20% of the cases. 99.50% of patients used NSAID, while glucosamine was used by 8.80%, prednisone by 4.90%, methotrexate by 3.40%, and relaxon by 4.40%. The number of fat injection was single in 97.10%, twice in 2.4%, or triple in 0.50% of cases (**Table 5**).

VAS values were significantly higher in preinjection versus postinjection both during rest (8.02 ± 1.81 versus 0.69 ± 0.64, $p < 0.0001$) and with activity (9.53 ± 0.88 versus 1.46 ± 0.80, $p < 0.0001$) which reflected a highly significant improvement in OA pain (**Table 6** and **Figure 3**).

Table 7 presented the Western Ontario and McMaster Universities Osteoarthritis Index before and after intra-articular fat micrograft injection. The three domains of WOMAC index, pain, stiffness, and physical function, were significantly lower in the post intra-articular fat injection period than the preinjection values. The total score of WOMAC test and its percentage were significantly lower in the post intra-articular fat injection period than the preinjection values (77.65 ± 11.84 versus 5.69 ± 4.60, $p < 0.0001$; 80.89 ± 12.34 versus 5.93 ± 4.79, $p < 0.0001$) (**Table 7** and **Figures 4–7**).

Visual analogue scale	Preinjection	Postinjection	Significance (*P*-value)
Rest	8.02 ± 1.81 (2.00–10.00)	0.69 ± 0.64 (0.00–4.00)	**0.0001**
Exercise	9.53 ± 0.88 (6.00–10.00)	1.46 ± 0.80 (0.00–5.00)	**0.0001**

Table 6.
Visual analogue scale values at rest and with activity before and after intra-articular fat micrograft injection.

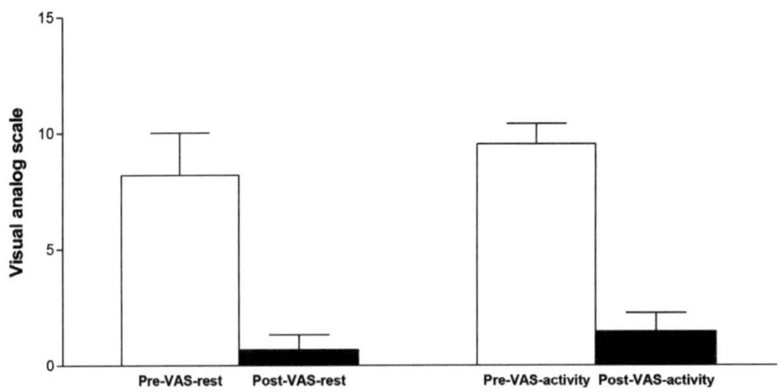

Figure 3.
Visual analogue scale values at rest and with activity before and after intra-articular fat micrograft injection.

Western Ontario and McMaster Universities Osteoarthritis Index	Preinjection	Postinjection	Significance (*P*-value)
Pain			
1. Walking	3.85 ± 0.401 (2.00–4.00)	0.65 ± 0.52 (0.00–2.00)	**0.0001**
2. Stair climbing	3.95 ± 0.24 (2.00–4.00)	0.98 ± 0.40 (0.00–2.00)	**0.0001**
3. Nocturnal	3.36 ± 0.76 (0.00–4.00)	0.25 ± 0.50 (0.00–4.00)	**0.0001**
4. Rest	3.15 ± 0.79 (0.00–4.00)	0.11 ± 0.32 (0.00–1.00)	**0.0001**
5. Weight-bearing	3.94 ± 0.29 (2.00–5.00)	0.96 ± 0.45 (0.00–2.00)	**0.0001**
Stiffness			
6. Morning stiffness	3.103 ± 0.89 (0.00–4.00)	0.20 ± 0.40 (0.00–1.00)	**0.0001**

Western Ontario and McMaster Universities Osteoarthritis Index	Preinjection	Postinjection	Significance (*P*-value)
7. Stiffness occurring later in the day	2.04 ± 1.17 (0.00–4.00)	0.14 ± 0.35 (0.00–1.00)	**0.0001**
Physical function			
8. Descending stairs	3.90 ± 0.34 (2.00–4.00)	0.93 ± 0.36 (0.00–2.00)	**0.0001**
9. Ascending stairs	3.92 ± 0.32 (2.00–4.00)	0.94 ± 0.45 (0.00–4.00)	**0.0001**
10. Rising from sitting	3.28 ± 0.76 (1.00–4.00)	0.20 ± 0.47 (0.00–4.00)	**0.0001**
11. Standing	3.52 ± 0.69 (1.00–4.00)	0.47 ± 0.58 (0.00–4.00)	**0.0001**
12. Bending to floor	3.09 ± 0.86 (0.00–4.00)	0.22 ± 0.43 (0.00–2.00)	**0.0001**
13. Walking on flat surface	3.20 ± 0.75 (1.00–4.00)	0.21 ± 0.41 (0.00–1.00)	**0.0001**
14. Getting in/out of car	3.40 ± 0.80 (1.00–4.00)	0.64 ± 0.54 (0.00–2.00)	**0.0001**
15. Going shopping	3.87 ± 0.41 (2.00–4.00)	1.02 ± 0.52 (0.00–2.00)	**0.0001**
16. Putting on socks	2.62 ± 0.84 (0.00–4.00)	0.22 ± 0.41 (0.00–1.00)	**0.0001**
17. Lying in bed	2.80 ± 0.91 (0.00–4.00)	0.12 ± 0.32 (0.00–1.00)	**0.0001**
18. Taking off socks	2.16 ± 0.86 (0.00–4.00)	0.05 ± 0.22 (0.00–1.00)	**0.0001**
19. Rising from bed	2.86 ± 0.86 (0.00–4.00)	0.14 ± 0.34 (0.00–1.00)	**0.0001**
20. Getting in/out of bath	3.84 ± 0.60 (0.00–4.00)	1.17 ± 0.60 (0.00–2.00)	**0.0001**
21. Sitting	2.95 ± 0.78 (0.00–4.00)	0.14 ± 0.40 (0.00–3.00)	**0.0001**
22. Getting on/off toilet	2.65 ± 0.79 (1.00–4.00)	0.14 ± 0.36 (0.00–2.00)	**0.0001**
23. Heavy domestic duties	3.91 ± 0.40 (1.00–4.00)	1.15 ± 0.53 (0.00–4.00)	**0.0001**
24. Light domestic duties	2.35 ± 0.76 (0.00–4.00)	0.04 ± 0.22 (0.00–2.00)	**0.0001**
Total score			
Out of 96	77.65 ± 11.84 (32.00–96.00)	5.69 ± 4.60 (0.00–24.00)	**0.0001**
Percentage (%)	80.89 ± 12.34 (33.33–100.00)	5.93 ± 4.79 (0.00–25.25)	**0.0001**

The activities in each category are rated according to the following scale of difficulty: 0 = none; 1 = slight; 2 = moderate; 3 = very; 4 = extremely. Data are expressed as mean ± SD (minimum-maximum). Wilcoxon test for nonparametric variables was used to compare pre- to postinjection values.

Table 7.
The Western Ontario and McMaster Universities Osteoarthritis Index before and after intra-articular fat micrograft injection.

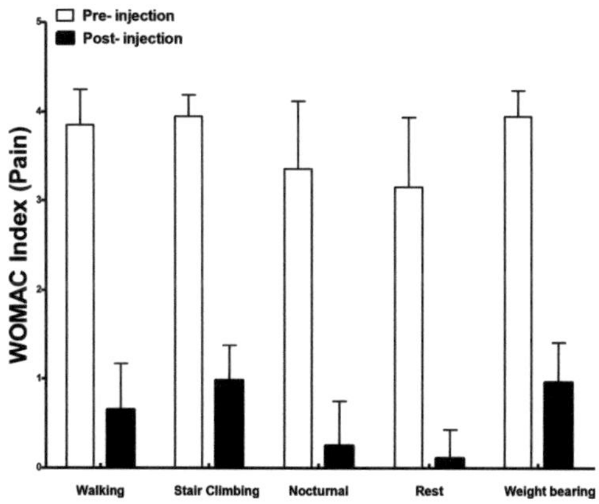

Figure 4.
The Western Ontario and McMaster Universities Osteoarthritis Index Pain before and after intra-articular fat micrograft injection.

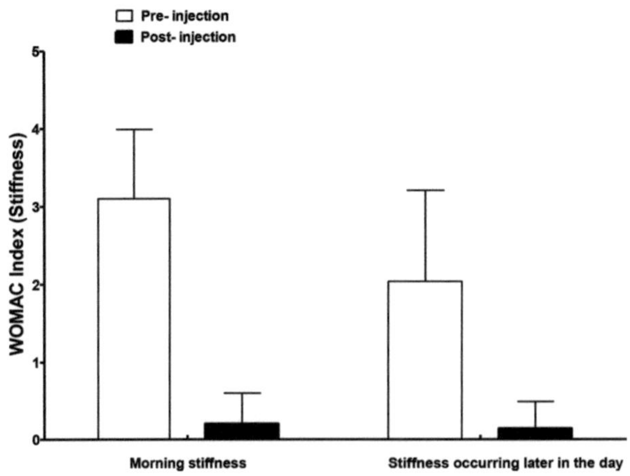

Figure 5.
The Western Ontario and McMaster Universities Osteoarthritis Index Stiffness before and after intra-articular fat micrograft injection.

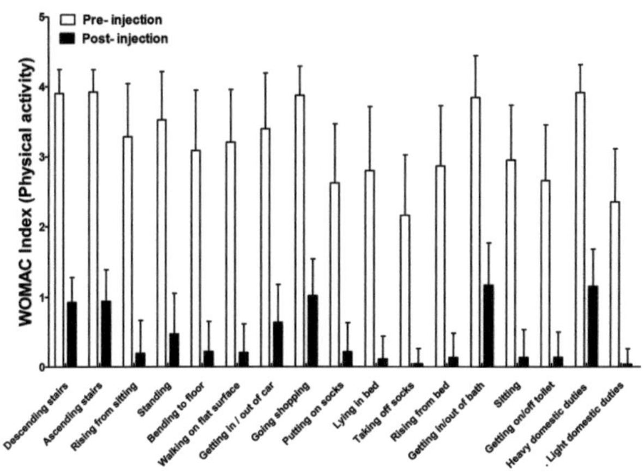

Figure 6.
The Western Ontario and McMaster Universities Osteoarthritis Index Physical activity before and after intra-articular fat micrograft injection.

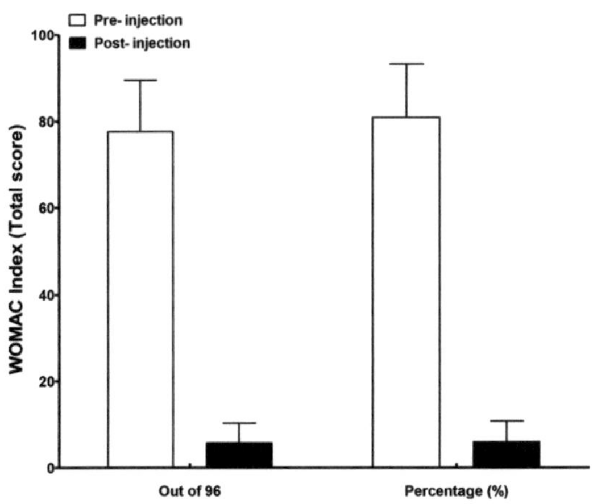

Figure 7.
The Western Ontario and McMaster Universities Osteoarthritis Index Total Score before and after intra-articular fat micrograft injection.

Wilcoxon test for nonparametric variables was used to compare pre- to postinjection values.

17. Complications

We did have complication like infection or graft rejection; it was well tolerated because it is autologous.

18. Conclusion

Over 10 years our clinical study of treatment of chronic osteoarthritis using intra-articular injection of autologous fat micrograft offers an effective and safe treatment as a nonantigenic, lubricating, regenerative, and reparative modality which helps to restore the damaged cartilages and in turn improve joint pain, mobility, and other functions of the osteoarthritic joints; it is minimally invasive, without scars, and with lower cost than other lines of therapy, improves the quality of life, and is mostly effective with single injection, but reinjection is needed in some patients according to disease severity and chronicity. We found a selection of patients and preoperative correction of risk factors, e.g., obesity muscle weakness led to better outcome of the procedure.

Conflict of interest

The authors have no conflict of interest.

Disclosure

The authors did not receive any type of commercial support either in forms of compensation or financial support for this study. The authors have no financial interest in any of the products or devices or drugs mentioned in this article.

Ethical approval

The study design was reviewed and approved by the Unit of Biomedical Ethics Research Committee at King Abdulaziz University.

Author details

Sabah S. Moshref[1*], Yasir S. Jamal[1], Amro M. Al-Hibshi[2] and Abdullah M. Kaki[3]

1 Department of Surgery, Faculty of Medicine, King Abdulaziz University Hospital, Jeddah, Saudi Arabia

2 Department of Orthopedics, Faculty of Medicine, King Abdulaziz University Hospital, Jeddah, Saudi Arabia

3 Department of Anesthesia and Critical Care, Faculty of Medicine, King Abdulaziz University Hospital, Jeddah, Saudi Arabia

*Address all correspondence to: dr.sabahmoshref@gmail.com

References

[1] Neuber G. Gustav Adolf Neuber (24 June 1850-13 April 1932) was a German surgeon born in Tondern (today-Tønder. Wir Kieler)

[2] Lexer E. Fettegewebe verpflanzung. In: Lexer E. Die freien Transplantation en. I Teil. Stuttgart: Enke; 1919. pp. 264-547

[3] Zuk PA, Zhu M, Mizuno H, Huang J, Futrell JW, Katz AJ, et al. Multilineage cells from human adipose tissue: Implications for cellbased therapies. Tissue Engineering. 2001;7:211-228

[4] Rigotti G, Marchi A, Galie M, Baroni G, Benati D, Krampera M, et al. Clinical treatment of radiotherapy tissue damage by lipoaspirate transplant: A healing process mediated by adipose-derived adult stem cells. Plastic and Reconstructive Surgery. 2007;**119**:1409-1422

[5] Liu Y, Wu J, Zhu Y, Han J. Therapeutic application of mesenchymal stem cells in bone and joint diseases. Clinical and Experimental Medicine. 2014;**14**(1): 13-24. DOI: 10.1007/s10238-012-0218-1. Epub: 3 November 2012 (Review)

[6] Moshref S, Jamal Y, Hummdi L, Kaki A, Al-Hibshi A. Intra-articular injection of autologous fat micro graft in sheep hind knee joints. Life Science Journal. 2013;**10**(4):2115-2120. (ISSN: 1545-1003). Available from: http://www.lifesciencesite.org. 281

[7] Moshref S, Kaki A, Al-Hibshi A, Jamal YS. Intra-articular injection of autologous fat micro-graft for the treatment of knee osteoarthritis: Preliminary experience. Life Science Journal. 2014;**11**(2):55-60

[8] Sun HB. Mechanical loading, cartilage degradation, and arthritis. Annals of the New York Academy of Sciences. 2010;**1211**:37-50

[9] The National Collaborating Centre for Chronic Conditions: Osteoarthritis. National clinical guideline for care and management in adults. Available from: www.nice.org.uk/nicemedia/pdf/CG59NICEguideline.pdf

[10] Goldring SR, Goldring MB. Bone and cartilage in osteoarthritis: Is what's best for one good or bad for the other? Arthritis Research and Therapy. 2011;**12**:143

[11] Aigner T, Rose J, Martin J, Buckwalter J. Aging theories of primary osteoarthritis: From epidemiology to molecular biology. Rejuvenation Research. 2004;**7**:134-145

[12] Mobasheri A. Applications of proteomics to osteoarthritis, a musculoskeletal disease characterized by aging. Frontiers in Physiology. 2011;**2**:108

[13] Gharbi M, Deberg M, Henrotin Y. Application for proteomic techniques in studying osteoarthritis: A review. Frontiers in Physiology. 2011;**2**:90

[14] Hunter DJ. Lower extremity osteoarthritis management needs a paradigm shift. British Journal of Sports Medicine. 2011;**45**:283-288

[15] Wilson DR, Mc Walter EJ, Johnston JD. The measurement of joint mechanics and their role in osteoarthritis genesis and progression. Rheumatic Diseases Clinics of North America. 2013;**39**(1):21-44. DOI: 10.1016/j.rdc.2012.11.002

[16] Schroeppel JP, Crist JD, Anderson HC, Wang J. Molecular regulation of articular chondrocyte function and its significance in osteoarthritis. Histology and Histopathology. 2011;**26**(3):377-394

[17] Chen FH, Tuan RS. Mesenchymal stem cells in arthritic diseases. Arthritis Research and Therapy. 2008;**10**(5):223

[18] Pendleton A, Arden N, Dougados M, et al. EULAR recommendations for the management of knee osteoarthritis: Report of a task force of the Standing Committee for International Clinical Studies Including Therapeutic Trials (ESCISIT). Annals of the Rheumatic Diseases. 2000;**59**(12):936-944

[19] Hernández-Díaz S, García-Rodríguez LA. Epidemiologic assessment of the safety of conventional nonsteroidal anti-inflammatory drugs. The American Journal of Medicine. 2001;**110**(Suppl 3):20S-27S

[20] Flood J. The role of acetaminophen in the treatment of osteoarthritis. The American Journal of Managed Care. 2010;**16**(Suppl Management):S48-S54

[21] Hameed F, Ihm J. Injectable medications for osteoarthritis. PM and R: The Journal of Injury, Function, and Rehabilitation. 2012;**4**(5 Suppl):S75-S81

[22] Miller LE, Block JE. US-approved intra-articular hyaluronic acid injections are safe and effective in patients with knee osteoarthritis: Systematic review and meta-analysis of randomized, saline-controlled trials. Clinical Medicine Insights: Arthritis and Musculoskeletal Disorders. 2013;**6**:57-63

[23] Rudzinski M. What Are Optimal Strategies in the Management of Osteoarthritis? Medscape Family Medicine. May 2001. Available at: http://www.medscape.com/viewarticle/413591 [Accessed: February 2016]

[24] Spaková T, Rosocha J, Lacko M, Harvanová D, Gharaibeh A. Treatment of knee joint osteoarthritis with autologous platelet-rich plasma in comparison with hyaluronic acid. American Journal of Physical Medicine & Rehabilitation. 2012;**91**(5):411-417

[25] Douleh D, Frank RM. Marrow stimulation: Microfracture, drilling, and abrasion. Operative Techniques in Sports Medicine. 2018;**26**(3):170-174

[26] Malchau H, Herberts P, Garellick G, Soderman P, Eisler T. Prognosis of total hip replacement: Update of results and risk-ratio analysis for revision and re-revision from the Swedish National Hip Arthoplasty Register 1979-2000. In: Scientific Exhibition. Presented at: 69th Annual Meeting of the American Academy of Orthopaedic Surgeons; 11-15 June 2002; Dallas, TX, USA

[27] Santaguida PL, Hawker GA, Hudak PL, et al. Patient characteristics affecting the prognosis of total hip and knee joint arthroplasty: A systematic review. Canadian Journal of Surgery. 2008;**51**(6):428-436

[28] Roberts S, Genever P, McCaskie A. Prospects of stem cell therapy in osteoarthritis. Regenerative Medicine. 2011;**6**(3):351-366. DOI: 10.2217/RME.11.21

[29] Vinatier C, Bouffi C, Merceron C, Gordeladze J, Brondello JM, Jorgensen C, et al. Cartilage tissue engineering: Towards a biomaterial-assisted mesenchymal stem cell therapy. Current Stem Cell Research & Therapy. 2009;**4**(4):318-329

[30] Oh W, Kim DS, Yang YS, Lee JK. Immunological properties of umbilical cord blood-derived mesenchymal stromal cells. Cellular Immunology. 2008;**251**:116-123

[31] Di Nicola M, Carlo-Stella C, Magni M, Milanesi M, Longoni PD, Matteucci P, et al. Human bone marrow stromal cells suppress T-lymphocyte proliferation induced by cellular or nonspecific mitogenic stimuli. Blood. 2002;**99**:3838-3843

[32] Ren G, Su J, Zhang L, Zhao X, Ling W, L'huillie A, et al. Species variation in the mechanisms of mesenchymall stem cell-mediated immunosuppression. Stem Cells. 2009;**27**:1954-1962

[33] Beyth S, Borovsky Z, Mevorach D, Liebergall M, Gazit Z, Aslan H, et al. Human mesenchymal stem cells alter antigen-presenting cell maturation and induced T-cell unresponsiveness. Blood. 2005;**105**:2214-2219

[34] Salibian AA, Widgerow AD, Abrouk M, Evans GRD. Stem cells in plastic surgery: A review of current clinical and translational applications. Archives of Plastic Surgery. 2013;**40**:666-675. Available from: http://dx.doi.org/10.5999/aps.2013.40.6.666 [Accepted: 25 September 2013] pISSN: 2234-6163, eISSN: 2234-6171

[35] Walia B, Satija N, Tripathi RP, et al. Induced pluripotent stem cells: Fundamentals and applications of the reprogramming process and its ramifications on regenerative medicine. Stem Cell Reviews. 2012;**8**:100-115

[36] Caplan AI, Dennis JE. Mesenchymal stem cells as trophic mediators. Journal of Cellular Biochemistry. 2006;**98**(5):1076-1084

[37] Lodi D, Iannitti T, Palmieri B. Stem cells in clinical practice: Applications and warnings. Journal of Experimental & Clinical Cancer Research. 2011;**30**:9

[38] Caplan AI. Review: Mesenchymal stem cells: Cell-based reconstructive therapy in orthopedics. Tissue Engineering. 2005;**11**(7-8):1198-1211

[39] da Silva ML, Chagatelles PC, Nardi NB. Mesenchymal stem cells reside in virtually all post-natal organs and tissues. Journal of Cell Science. 2006;**119**:2204-2213

[40] Campagnoli C, Roberts IA, Kumar S, Bennett PR, Bellantuono I, Fisk NM. Identification of mesenchymal stem/progenitor cells in human first-trimester fetal blood, liver, and bone marrow. Blood. 2001;**98**:2396-2402

[41] Kim JY, Jeon HB, Yang YS, Oh W, Chang JW. Application of human umbilical cord blood-derived mesenchymal stem cells in disease models. World Journal of Stem Cells. 2010;**2**:34-38

[42] Rodriguez AM, Elabd C, Amri EZ, Aihaud G, Dani C. The human adipose tissue is a source of multipotent stem cells. Biochimie. 2005;**87**:125-128

[43] Ilancheran S, Moodley Y, Manuelpillai U. Human fetal membranes: A source of stem cells for tissue regeneration and repair? Placenta. 2009;**30**:2-10

[44] Vishnubalaji R, Al-Nbaheen M, Kadalmani B, Aldahmash A, Ramesh T. Comparative investigation of the differentiation capability of bone-marrow-and adipose-derived mesenchymal stem cells by qualitative and quantitative analysis. Cell and Tissue Research. 2012;**347**:419-427

[45] Guilak F, Awad HA, Fermor B, Leddy HA, Gimble JM. Adipose derived adult stem cells for cartilage tissue engineering. Biorheology. 2004;**41**:389-399

[46] Murphy JM, Fink DJ, Hunziker EB, Barry FP. Stem cell therapy in a caprine model of osteoarthritis. Arthritis and Rheumatism. 2003;**48**:3464-3474

[47] Guo X, Wang X, Zhang Y, Xia R, Hu M, Duan C. Repair of large articular cartilage defects with implants of autologous mesenchymal stem cells seeded into beta-tricalcium phosphate in a sheep model. Tissue Engineering. 2004;**10**:1818-1829

[48] JHP H, Chen F, Thambyah A, Lee EH. Treatment of chondral lesions in advanced osteochondritis dissecans: a comparative study of the efficacy of chondrocytes, mesenchymal stem cells, periosteal graft, and mosaicplasty (osteochondral autograft) in animal models. Journal of Pediatric Orthopedics. 2004;**24**:427-433

[49] Liu Y, Shu XZ, Prestwich GD. Osteochondral defect repair with autologous bone marrow-derived mesenchymal stem cells in an injectable, in situ, cross-linked synthetic extracellular matrix. Tissue Engineering. 2006;**12**:3405-3416

[50] Kayakabe M, Tsutsumi S, Watanabe H, Kato Y, Takagishi K. Transplantation of autologous rabbit BM-derived mesenchymal stromal cells embedded in hyaluronic acid gel sponge into osteochondral defects of the knee. Cytotherapy. 2006;**8**:343-353

[51] Yan H, Yu C. Repair of full-thickness cartilage defects with cells of different origin in a rabbit model. Arthroscopy. 2007;**23**:178-187

[52] Lee KBL, Hui JHP, Song IC, Ardany L, Lee EH. Injectable mesenchymal stem cell therapy for large cartilage defects—A porcine model. Stem Cells. 2007;**25**:2964-2971

[53] Kuroda R, Ishida K, Matsumoto T, Akisue T, Fujioka H, Mizuno K. Treatment of a full-thickness articular cartilage defect in the femoral condyle of an athlete with autologous bone marrow stromal cells. Osteoarthritis and Cartilage. 2007;**15**:226-231

[54] Black LL, Gaynor J, Adams C, Dhupa S, Sams AE, Taylor R, et al. Effect of intraarticular injection of autologous adipose-derived mesenchymal stem and regenerative cells on clinical signs of chronic osteoarthritis of the elbow joint in dogs. Veterinary Therapeutics. 2008;**9**:192-200

[55] Black LL, Gaynor J, Gahring D, Adams C, Aron D, Harman S, et al. Effect of adipose-derived mesenchymal stem and regenerative cells on lameness in dogs with chronic osteoarthritis of the coxofemoral joints: A randomized, double-blinded, multicenter, controlled trial. Veterinary Therapeutics. 2007;**8**:272-284

[56] Noth U, Steinert AF, Tuan RS. Technology insight: Adult mesenchymal stem cells for osteoarthritis therapy: Delivery modes for mesenchymal stem cells. Nature Clinical Practice. Rheumatology. 2008;**4**:371-380

[57] Horie M, Sekiya I, Muneta T, Ichinose S, Matsumoto K, Saito H, et al. Intra-articular injected synovial stem cells differentiate into meniscal cells directly and promote meniscal regeneration without mobilization of distant organs in rat massive meniscal defect. Stem Cells. 2009;**27**:878-887

[58] Mokbel AN, El Tookhy OS, Shamaa AA, Rashed LA, Sabry D, El Sayed AM. Homing and reparative effect of intra-articular injection of autologous mesenchymal stem cells in osteoarthritic animal model. BMC Musculoskeletal skeletal Disorders. 2011;**12**:259

[59] Sato M, Uchida K, Nakajima H, Miyazaki T, Guerrero AR, Watanabe S, et al. Direct transplantation of mesenchymal stem cells into the knee joints of Hartley strain guinea pigs with spontaneous osteoarthritis. Arthritis Research and Therapy. 2012;**14**:R31

[60] Ameye LG, Young MF. Animal models of osteoarthritis: Lessons learned while seeking the 'Holy Grail'. Current Opinion in Rheumatology. 2006;**18**:537-547

[61] Desando G, Cavallo C, Sartoni F, Martini L, Parrilli A, Veronesi F, et al. Intra-articular delivery of adipose derived stromal cells attenuates osteoarthritis progression in an experimental rabbit model. Arthritis Research and Therapy. 2013;**15**:R22. DOI: 10.1186/ar4156

[62] van Lent PLEM, van den Berg WB. Mesenchymal stem cell therapy in osteoarthritis: Advanced tissue repair or intervention with smouldering synovial activation? Arthritis Research and Therapy. 2013;**15**:112

[63] Hou T, Xu J, Wu X, Xie Z, Luo F, Zhang Z, et al. Umbilical cord Wharton's Jelly: A new potential cell source of mesenchymal stromal cells for bone tissue engineering. Tissue Engineering. Part A. 2009;**15**:2325-2334

[64] Fan CG, Zhang Q J, Zhou JR. Therapeutic potentials of mesenchymal stem cells derived from human umbilical cord. Stem Cell Reviews. 2011;7:195-207

[65] Fong CY, Subramanian A, Gauthaman K, Venugopal J, Biswas A, Ramakrishna S, et al. Human umbilical cord Wharton's Jelly stem cells undergo enhanced chondrogenic differentiation when grown on nanofibrous scaffolds and in a sequential two-stage culture medium environment. Stem Cell Reviews. 2012;**8**:195-209

[66] Moshref S, Jamal S, Al-Hibshi A, Kaki A. Intra-articular injection of autologous fat graft for the treatment of knee osteoarthritis. Life Science Journal. 2017;**14**(4):30-35. DOI: 10.7537/marslsj140417.05. ISSN: 1097-8135 (Print)/ISSN: 2372-613X (Online). Available from: http://www.lifesciencesite.com

[67] Kon E, Filardo G, Roffi A, Andriolo L, Marcacci M. New trends for knee cartilage regeneration: From cell-free scaffolds to mesenchymal stem cells. Current Reviews in Musculoskeletal Medicine. 2012;**5**(3, 243):236

[68] Madry H, Grun UW, Knutsen G. Cartilage repair and joint preservation: Medical and surgical treatment options. Deutsches Arzteblatt International Impact Factor. 2011;**108**(40):669-677

[69] Filardo G, Madry H, Jelic M, Roffi A, Cucchiarini M, Kon E. Mesenchymal stem cells for the treatment of cartilage lesions: From preclinical findings to clinical application in orthopaedics. Knee Surgery, Sports Traumatology, Arthroscopy. 2013;**21**:1717-1729. DOI: 10.1007/s00167-012-2329-3

[70] Wakitani S, Imoto K, Yamamoto T, Saito M, Murata N, Yoneda M. Human autologous culture expanded bone marrow mesenchymal cell transplantation for repair of cartilage defects in osteoarthritic knee. Osteoarthritis and Cartilage. 2002;**10**:199-206

[71] Ohgushi H, Kotobuki N, Funaoka H, Machida H, Hirose M, Tanaka Y, et al. Tissue engineered ceramic artificial joint—Ex vivo osteogenic differentiation of patient mesenchymal cells on total ankle joints for treatment of osteoarthritis. Biomaterials. 2005;**26**:4654-4661

[72] Centeno CJ, Busse D, Kisiday J, Keohan C, Freeman M, Karli D. Increased knee cartilage volume in degenerative joint disease using percutaneously implanted, autologous mesenchymal stem cells. Pain Physician. 2008;**11**:343-353

[73] Buda R, Vannini F, Cavallo M, Grigolo B, Cenacchi A, Giannini S. Osteochondral lesions of the knee: A new one-step repair technique with bone-marrow-derived cells. The Journal of Bone and Joint Surgery American Volume. 2010;**92**(Suppl 2):2-11

[74] Pak J. Regeneration of human bones in hip osteonecrosis and human cartilage in knee osteoarthritis with autologous adipose-tissue-derived stem cells: A case series. Journal of Medical Case Reports. 2011;**5**:296

[75] Koh YG, Choi YJ. Infrapatellar fat pad-derived mesenchymal stem cell therapy for knee osteoarthritis. The Knee. 2012;**19**(6):902-907

[76] Davatchi F, Abdollahi BS, Mohyeddin M, Shahram F, Nikbin B. Mesenchymal stem cell therapy for knee

osteoarthritis. Preliminary report of four patients. International Journal of Rheumatic Diseases. 2011;**14**:211-215

[77] Koh YG, Jo SB, Kwon OR, Suh DS, Lee SW, Park SH, et al. Mesenchymal stem cell injections improve symptoms of knee osteoarthritis. Arthroscopy: The Journal of Arthroscopic and Related Surgery: Official Publication of the Arthroscopy Association of North America and the International Arthroscopy Association. 2013;**29**(4):748-755

[78] Koh YG, Choi YJ, Kwon SK, Kim YS, Yeo JE. Clinical results and second-look arthroscopic findings after treatment with adipose-derived stem cells for knee osteoarthritis. Knee Surgery, Sports Traumatology, Arthroscopy. 2015;**23**(5):1308-1313

Chapter 6

High Tibial Osteotomy

Tuna Pehlivanoglu, Kerem Yildirim and Tahsin Beyzadeoglu

Abstract

To address lower limb malalignment with concomitant medial compartment osteoarthritis, meniscal deficiency, focal chondral defects, and ligamentous instability, high tibia osteotomy (HTO) is a reliable treatment option. In order to achieve a good long-term outcome with HTO, a comprehensive history and physical examination, together with a meticulous patient selection and careful pre-operative planning, and selection of the appropriate fixation technique and rehabilitation protocol are paramount.

Keywords: medial compartment osteoarthritis, chondral defect, high tibial osteotomy, medial opening wedge, lateral closing wedge, survival rates, complications

1. Introduction

Cartilage degeneration of a particular compartment of the knee joint is usually the result of overloading of medial compartment which is associated with the malalignment of the lower extremity. In other words, cartilage degeneration is an inevitable result of lower extremity malalignment and it is associated with clinical symptoms including pain and gait difficulty. In addition to arthritis, rickets, Blount disease, or tibial plateau fractures are other reasons for lower limb deformity, but we will not further mention them here because they are irrelevant to this chapter. In order to prevent the progressive cartilage degeneration followed by amelioration of the symptoms, re-alignment osteotomies, which have the potential to unload the compartment while preserving the native joint, are generally applied. Considering the relative young age of these patients with unicompartmental arthrosis, in order to delay the arthroplasty, re-alignment osteotomies, while being technically challenging constitute the most important treatment modality by providing earlier return to high-level activities in contrast to arthroplasty. Osteotomies might also be applied with procedures including meniscal repairs, ligamentous reconstructions, or cartilage regenerating procedures, because of augmenting the success rates of these co-applied procedures. Indications for re-alignment osteotomies have been expanded recently as a result of high activity levels of the relatively older patients. Meanwhile, an optimization of the re-alignment osteotomies occurred as a result of the modified surgical instruments and techniques, leading to more reliable outcomes.

In young and active patients, it is important to preserve the medial compartment of the knee and provide adequate cartilage coverage to prevent a premature arthritis and to delay the arthroplasty as much as possible [1]. High tibial osteotomy (HTO) for varus deformity is one of the most common types of osteotomies for the re-alignment of the knee.

First HTO was performed by Jackson and Waugh in 1958, while they defined the technique as a ball and socket osteotomy inferior to anterior tibial tuberosity and at the middle third portion of the fibula [2]. Modifications of the original technique were reported with a success rate of 85% [3]. In 1965, Coventry reported his results regarding long-term outcomes, which was not very promising and made several publications in the following years [4]. The introduction of the blade plate for maintaining correction and allowing early motion was undertaken by Koshino. Opening wedge technique was later introduced by Hernigou and Debeyre with medial approach, where bone grafts and plates were used in order to have a stable fixation, while they recognized the importance of maintaining the sagittal slope while the coronal plane was being corrected [5, 6]. In the beginning of 1980, Maquet described the tibial dome osteotomy. The modern HTO is actually a variation of the Coventry osteotomy. HTO's high popularity between 1960 and 1980, showed a slow decline afterwards as a result of many reported good outcomes of total-unicondylar knee arthroplasty that changed the surgeons' preferences.

HTO is regaining popularity, especially in young and active patients with high expectations for physical activities and increased life expectancy, in order to preserve the native joint together with bone stock, cartilage covering and proprioception, which are compromised with unicompartmental knee arthroplasty, in addition to its allowance to relatively limited physical activities [1, 7, 8]. The currently used plates are providing very stable osteosynthesis by preserving the periosteal blood supply; while there are also new biomaterials and bone substitutes that prevent many complications related to iliac crest graft harvest [9–11]. Meanwhile, HTO became a more popular option for young and active patients as a result of the improvements regarding the surgical technique, fixation devices, and fewer complications accompanied with a meticulous patient selection [12–15].

HTO, as a re-alignment osteotomy is applied to transfer the medially deviated mechanical axis to lateral toward the midline of the knee to unload the medial compartment and delay the process of osteoarthritis (OA) [11, 13, 14]. The first aim of HTO is to eliminate or reduce pain, by translating loads to the contralateral (femorotibial) compartment as a result of the deformity correction; while some studies has reported that the regenerative process was beginning after the accomplishment of re-alignment [16–18].

2. Indications

Careful pre-operative planning and strict indication criteria are paramount in order to have a successful outcome in the long term [1, 11].

Indications of HTO can be categorized as physical and radiological. Physical indications include: *an age between 40 and 70 years; a well-localized pain at the medial joint line; an arc of flexion more than 90° and, a lack of extension less than 10°; normal or correctable ligamentous status, while anterior cruciate ligament [ACL] or posterior cruciate ligament [PCL] insufficiency is not a contraindication; non-reducible deformity; and an active lifestyle* [7, 11].

Physical contraindications comprise: *any inflammatory disease, obesity, smoking, history of meniscectomy in the contralateral compartment, osteoarthritis in the contralateral compartment, and a tibial subluxation more than 1 cm.*

Radiological indications include: *no contralateral femorotibial joint space narrowing or patellofemoral joint space narrowing, partial or complete joint space narrowing in one compartment, significant symptomatic chondral injury to the patellofemoral or lateral compartments, tricompartmental arthritis and extra-articular deformity more than 5°* [1, 14]. To accurately assess the lateral compartment MRI could be very helpful.

Controversial contraindications regarding the HTO procedure include: *age > 60; obese females; flexion less than 120°, flexion contracture > 5°, or fixed flexion deformity; patellofemoral arthritis; accompanying severe extra-articular deformity* [11, 14].

HTO was recently suggested to be included in joint preservation surgery, to unload a cartilage restoration site (autologous chondrocyte implantation [ACI], osteochondral autograft or allograft, microfracture), and to correct the sagittal slope in cruciate ligament insufficiency [1, 8, 17]. When HTO is performed before medial compartment, arthritis has become severe and subchondral bone has been exposed, superior clinical and outcomes can be achieved [19, 20].

We would like to underline some important scenarios that should be meticulously assessed. Patients with anterior knee pain may get worse after the HTO procedure providing a coronal plane correction that can worsen their symptoms. Patients should be carefully explained, that the recovery from an HTO is time consuming and requiring commitment of the patient. Patients should be explained, that HTO procedure's post-operative rehabilitation protocol typically requires a period of protected weight-bearing followed by extensive lower limb muscular training. Patients should understand that an average of 6 months is needed to have a total recovery to a pain-free state of full activity. It is also very important that, pre-operatively, patient expectations should be thoroughly discussed and managed appropriately.

Indications of HTO might differ according to the geographical region. Patients older than 60 of age are typically offered total or unicompartmental knee arthroplasty over an HTO in the United States, while outside the United States, HTO is frequently performed in older patients, who are fit and active, and are explained that they may not obtain total symptom relief [1, 8].

It should be noted that the ideal patient for the application of HTO is a relatively young, active, and non-smoking patient, for whom arthroplasty should be prevented or delayed. As described above, obesity was also reported as a contraindication in old patients, because of the increased stresses that the osteotomy site must support; while it is a relative indication in younger patients in whom arthroplasty is indicated [1, 8].

A large-scale population-based study looking at 2671 patients who had undergone an HTO before conversion to a TKA found that certain factors lowered HTO survival rates, including accompanied ligament injuries, prior meniscectomy, older age, and female sex were reported to lower the HTO survival rates in 2761 patients, who underwent HTO before conversion to total knee arthroplasty [21].

3. Patient history and physical exam

A thorough history and physical exam are paramount before proceeding with HTO. As a result of that, patients with a prior traumatic knee injury and patients with a new onset of medial compartment arthritis could be distinguished. Previous trauma may be associated with other concomitant ligamentous and cartilaginous injuries. In every patient, in order to meet the expectations, the levels of activity, and overall health should be precisely noted.

Physical exam starts with the observation of patient's gait and stance, especially to assess varus thrust, accompanied with the presence of lateral collateral ligament insufficiency. Patients with varus deformity at the knee joint can be identified by observing them standing and walking. However, in cases of large body habitus, observation alone might not be very reliable. Examination of gait is critical regarding the decision with HTO. In patients with varus deformity at the knee joint, medial compartment is overloaded which creates an increased knee adduction moment, leading to increased stresses of the tensions of lateral ligamentous structures. In the presence of varus malalignment at knee joint, lateral ligamentous insufficiency may develop over time, and can even progress to varus recurvatum deformity associated with anterior cruciate ligament (ACL) insufficiency requiring ligament reconstruction in addition to HTO procedure [1, 11]. Joint instability including insufficiency of collateral and cruciate ligaments, any ankle deformity and limb length discrepancy should be considered for concomitant or staged surgery [22, 23].

4. Radiographic evaluation

A complete radiographic evaluation comprises the following X-rays:

- A full-length, three-joint (bilateral hip to ankle on the same cassette) weight-bearing view in full extension with the feet in a neutral position to evaluate the alignment;

- A 45° flexion posteroanterior view to evaluate any narrowing in the posterior femorotibial compartment;

- A lateral view to measure patellar height and assess the patellofemoral joint (PFJ);

- Stress views are mandatory when physical exam reveals ligamentous laxity,

- The tibia bone varus angle (TBVA) is measured on AP radiograph and TBVA > 5° is a good prognostic factor after osteotomy

- A skyline view for detailed evaluation of the patellofemoral joint [1, 8, 11].

Indices regarding the pre-operative patellar height (Caton-Deschamps index, modified Insall-Salvati index, Blackburne-Peel index) should be calculated because both opening and closing wedge HTOs have had the potential to result in patella baja. Therefore, patients with pre-existing patella baja should be evaluated very carefully before performing the HTO procedure [24, 25].

To establish the posterior tibial slope baseline, a lateral radiograph should be obtained. Because of the anatomical-triangular shape of tibia, a medial opening wedge osteotomy comprises a bone cut from anteromedial to posterolateral aspect of the tibia. As the osteotomy site is opened, the tibial slope increases. For a lateral closing wedge osteotomy, the same principle can be used but in a reverse fashion. Considering this type of osteotomy, the bone cut is directed from anterolateral-to-posteromedial, decreasing the tibial slope [1, 23].

In knee joints with cruciate ligament deficiencies, tibial slope changes could directly affect the problem regarding the ligaments. Meanwhile, PCL insufficiency is accentuated by an increased tibial slope, while in an ACL-deficient knee as a result of the decreased tibial slope, the degree of instability is frequently progressed [1, 21, 24]. However, to improve the outcome of HTO procedure, tibial slope adjustments can be applied. To enhance stability in an ACL-deficient knee, tibial slope may be increased, whereas in PCL-deficient knees decreasing the slope can be helpful in establishing stability [1, 21, 24]. We recommend using magnetic resonance imaging (MRI) in order to evaluate the soft tissue problems, including meniscus tears, ligamentoıus injuries, osteochondral defects, or even for the detection of subchondral bone edema.

5. Patient selection

In 2004, ISAKOS (International Society of Arthroscopy, Knee Surgery and Orthopedic Sports Medicine) developed a protocol for the HTO [23]. As a result of that protocol, an ideal patient for HTO is defined by following criteria:

- Malalignment < 15°
- Metaphyseal varus (i.e., TBVA > 5°)
- Full range of motion (ROM) of the knee joint
- Normal, near-normal lateral, and patellofemoral compartments
- No ligamentous instability
- Non-smoker
- Moderately active high-demand patient
- Young (40–60 years of age)
- BMI < 30 (in other words: obesity is a contraindication)
- Isolated medial joint line tenderness
- Some level of pain tolerance

HTO is contraindicated in patients with followings:

- Severe OA of the medial compartment (Ahlback grade III or higher)
- Tricompartmental OA
- Patellofemoral OA
- Age > 65
- Knee ROM < 120°
- Knee flexion contracture > 5°
- Diagnosis of inflammatory arthritis
- Heavy smokers
- large area of exposed bone on tibial and femoral articular surface (>15 × 15 mm)

Good prognostic factors [26–28] regarding the HTO procedure can be summarized as the followings:

- Ahlback grade 0 arthritis of medial plateau

- Age < 50
- Pre-operative TBVA > 5°
- Post-operative obliquity of tibiofemoral joint line in a narrow range close to 0°
- Anatomical valgus alignment of ≥8° at 5 weeks post-op
- Excellent pre-operative Knee Society Score (KSS)

Poor prognostic factors [26–28] regarding the HTO procedure can be summarized as the followings:

- Smoking
- Obesity
- Age > 56 years
- Valgus alignment of ≤5° at 5 weeks post-op
- Post-operative flexion < 120°

Cartilage defect at the medial tibial plateau was shown not to affect the clinical results of HTO procedure by Niemeyer et al. [14] in their study with minimum of 36-month follow-up of 69 patients after medial open wedge high tibial osteotomy (MOWHTO). They also concluded that partial thickness defect in lateral tibial plateau was well-tolerated.

6. Pre-operative decision-making and planning

Before starting with the decision-making process, some important terms regarding the alignment of the lower extremities should be explained [29–32].

- **Mechanical axis:** A line drawn from the center of the femoral head to the center of the knee.
- **Anatomical axis:** A line drawn from the piriformis fossa to the center of the knee joint and a line through the long axis of the tibia.
- **Weight-bearing axis:** A line drawn from the center of the femoral head to the center of ankle joint.

Normal values of the aforementioned axis are [29–32]:

- **Mechanical axis:** 1–3° varus
- **Anatomical axis:** 5–7° valgus
- 6° of valgus between the mechanical and anatomical axes

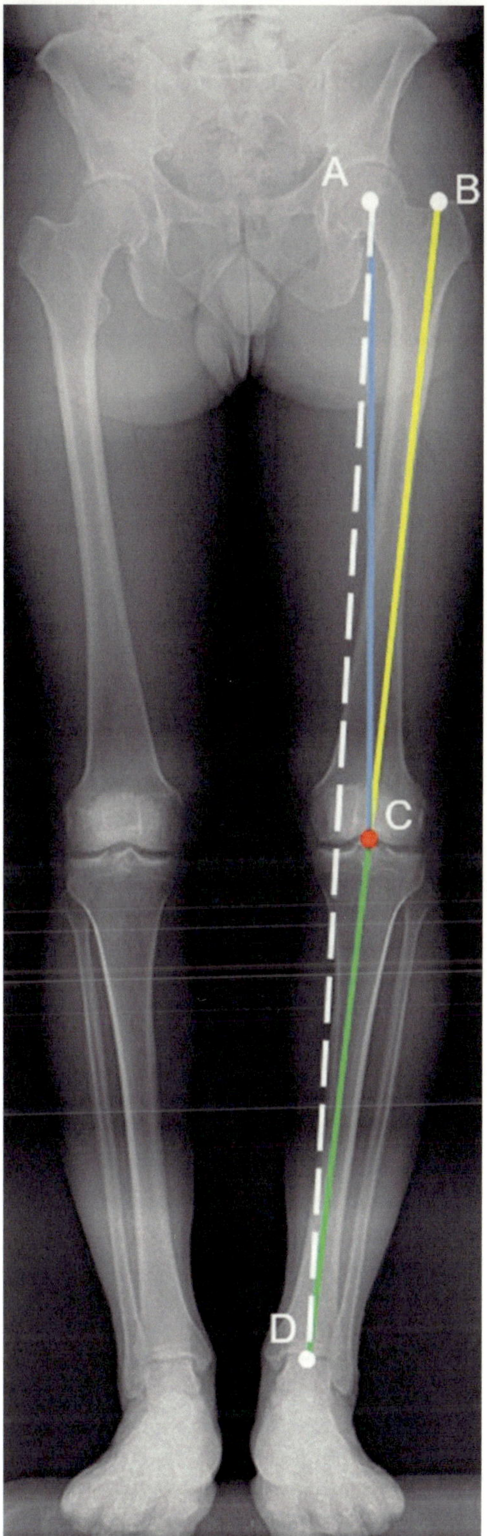

Figure 1.
The main axes of the lower extremity. AC: mechanical axis of femur, BC: anatomical axis of femur, CD: anatomical and mechanical axis of tibia, and AD: weight-bearing axis.

- Weight-bearing line passing through the lateral 30–40% of the tibial plateau
- 60% of the total body weight force passes through the medial compartment.

These measurements are performed on the alignment view (**Figure 1**). As a result of that, the type, location, and most importantly the amount of corrective osteotomy is ascertained. The pre-operative mechanical axis deviation and the degree of medial compartment arthrosis determine the amount of correction needed. Unicompartmental OA was reported to yield clinical symptoms, when the lower extremity alignment was a more than 10° of normal range [33].

If a decision to perform the HTO procedure is established, a medial opening wedge osteotomy or a lateral closing wedge osteotomy can be chosen purely based on the surgeon's decision.

Lateral closing wedge osteotomy, which allow for immediate weight-bearing, possess lower rates of non-union/mal-union, and is theoretically associated with lower risks of increasing the posterior sagittal slope and leading to patella baja was widely used by Coventry in 1960s [34, 35]. However, an exposure violating the anterior compartment of the leg, loss of the present bone stock together with a narrow window for modification once the bone wedge is removed, a possible concomitant fibular osteotomy, and risks associated with peroneal nerve exposure are the disadvantages associated with lateral closing wedge osteotomy.

Recently, as a result of advancements regarding low-contact profile-plated and fixation techniques, bone grafting options and most importantly regarding the technical advantages of the exposure and approach, medial opening wedge osteotomy has gained popularity [10, 13, 14]. By performing the HTO from the medial side and avoiding the lateral side, certain risks associated with the anterior compartment dissection, peroneal nerve exploration and fibular osteotomies can be avoided [8, 13, 14]. HTO procedure, performed as medial opening wedge osteotomy, facilitates correction and allow for fine-tuning in both the coronal and the sagittal planes. However, the risk to increase the sagittal slope and historically higher rates of non-union are the associated disadvantages of this approach [36].

7. Pre-operative planning of correction

The degree of correction is established according to the location of the mechanical axis line through the knee joint [1, 8]. The reference point on the tibial plateau is set at 62.5% of its width as measured from the medial cortex for most cases of genu varum resulting from OA [1, 14, 32]. In order to unload the medial compartment, the mechanical axis is planned to pass lateral to the center of the knee, aiming the lateral compartment [1, 14, 32] (**Figure 2**). A careful pre-operative planning should be undertaken in order to avoid the overloading of the lateral compartment, especially in cases with mild degenerative changes within the lateral compartment [14, 21, 36]. In these cases, massive corrections, or subtle corrections with a concomitant cartilage transplant, the mechanical axis can be moved to the midline of the knee joint to prevent overloading of the lateral side [14, 21, 36].

HTO procedure aims to reach a slight valgus axis to prevent any recurring of genu varum deformity. 3–5° of valgus in the mechanical axis or 8–10° of valgus in the anatomical axis are considered as the primary goals regarding correction after surgery [1, 5, 16, 34]. There is a fine balance between over- and under-correction; while slight varus correction can lead to recurrence of previous deformity, whereas overcorrection and over-deviation of the axis to the lateral compartment

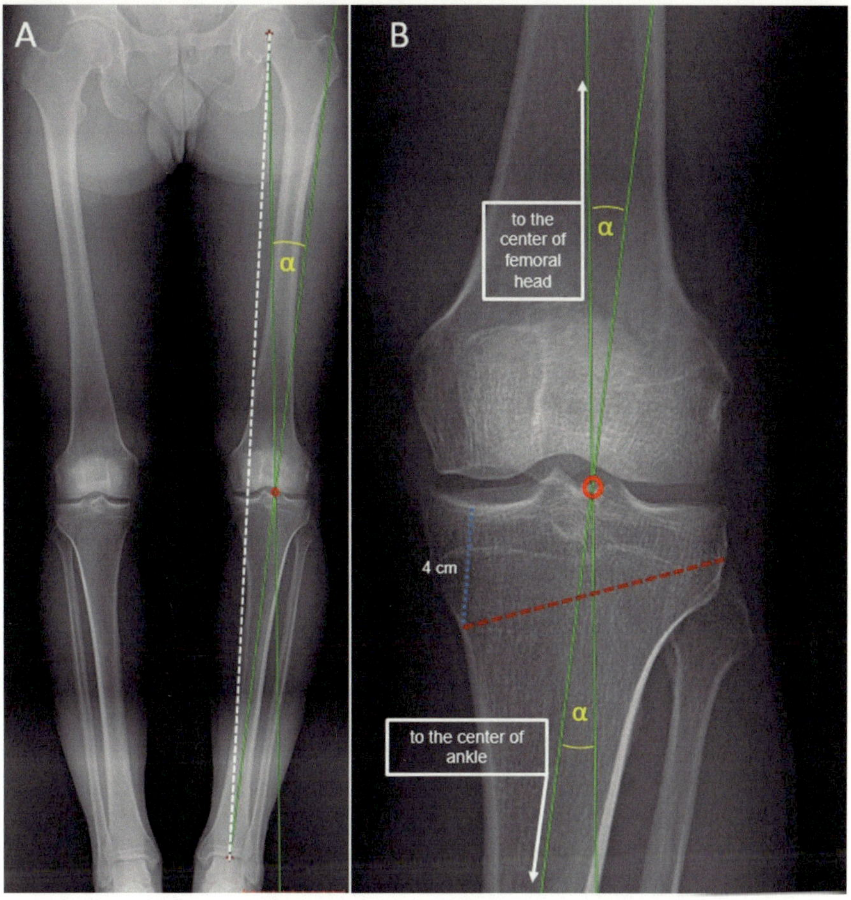

Figure 2.
Pre-operative planning for MOWHTO. (A) The white dashed line represents the weight-bearing axis, whereas the red circle represents the desired point where the weight-bearing axis is planned to pass post-operatively. (B) α, the correction angle, is the angle formed by the mechanical axes of femur and tibia that are aimed to be provided post-operatively. The osteotomy line (the red dashed line) is planned to be started about 4 cm distal to the medial joint line, aiming the tip of the head of fibula.

can cause cartilage degeneration at the lateral compartment, leading to lateral compartment OA [1, 5, 16, 34].

The weight-bearing line (WBL) should pass from 62% of the tibial plateau width when measured from the medial edge point of the medial tibial plateau [32, 37]. The point where WBL intersects the tibial plateau is called as the Fujisawa point [32, 37] (**Figure 3**). Fujisawa point is located slightly lateral to the lateral tibial spine and matches over the mechanical axis with 3–5° of valgus [32, 37]. A line is drawn from this point to the center of the ankle joint and another line from this point to the center of the ipsilateral femoral head is drawn to determine the amount of required correction [32, 37]. The angle measured between these two lines indicates the amount of required correction to re-align the knee joint [11, 32, 37]. The line for the osteotomy is drawn approximately 4 cm below the medial joint line toward the fibular head. This line has to be transferred to the apex of triangle that is created just during planning. The width of the triangle's base corresponds to the amount of correction that is required during a medial open wedge osteotomy [11, 13, 14].

The correction angle for lateral closing wedge osteotomies is calculated using a similar technique. Perpendicular to the axis of tibia and approximately 2 cm below

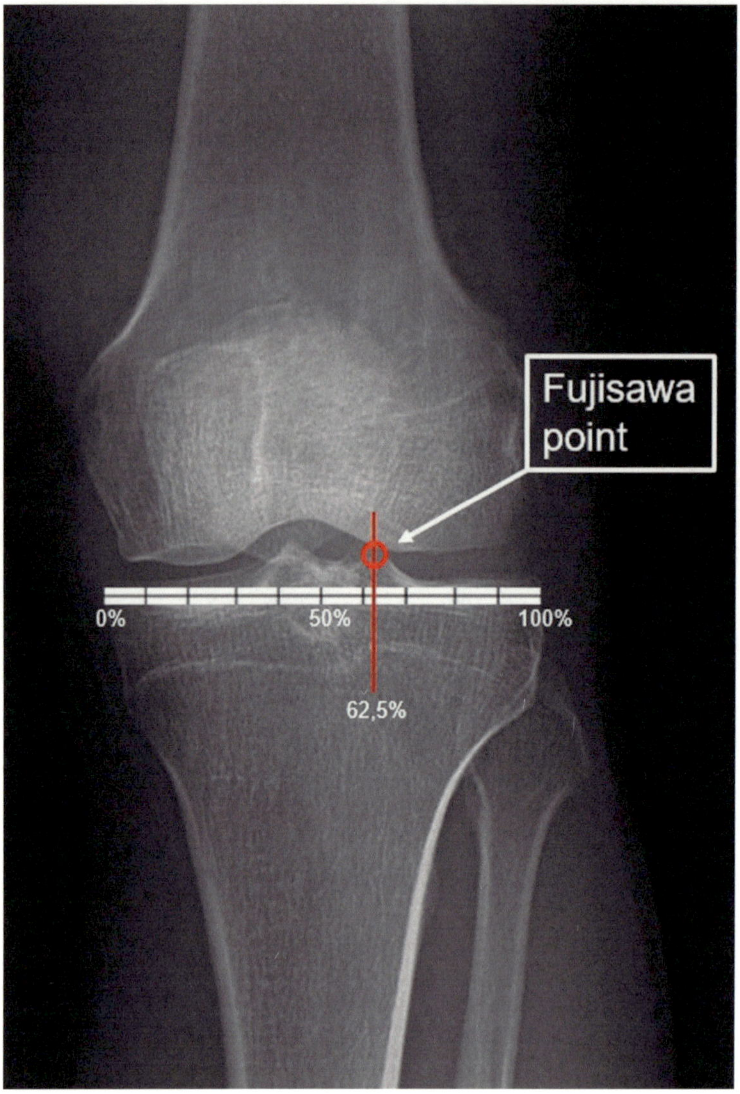

Figure 3.
Picture defining Fujisawa point.

the joint line the first osteotomy line is drawn. Applying the 1° to 1-mm equivalence at the lateral cortex below the initial osteotomy, the second osteotomy line is drawn. The wedge that has been bordered by the two osteotomy lines should be removed. By performing lateral closing wedge osteotomies, the sagittal slope must be assessed repeatedly to avoid significant slope perturbations [5, 8, 12].

8. Surgical technique

We usually start with arthroscopy to perform the debridement of the lateral compartment and to manage the concomitant pathologies regarding the menisci and chondral tissues before starting with the HTO, as recommended [38]. For the correction of genu varum deformity and re-alignment of the lower extremity, medial opening wedge, lateral closing wedge, and dome osteotomy can safely be applied. Our preference is the medial opening wedge osteotomy.

8.1 Medial open wedge osteotomy

In the middle of the line drawn from the tibial tubercule to medial border of tibia, a 3–5 cm longitudinal skin incision is made carefully by beginning 1–2 cm inferior to the medial joint line and continuing caudally to the pes anserinus. After dividing the sartorial fascia, we usually distract the tendons of pes anserinus distally, but an inverted L-shaped flap can also be elevated. After subperiosteal dissection and sufficient exposure of the proximal-medial tibia and the joint line, the superficial medial collateral ligament (sMCL) fibers are elevated from their medial tibial attachment sides; otherwise, if the attachment of sMCL is left intact on the medial tibia, pressures of the medial compartment may inevitably increase as a result of the tensioning of sMCL fibers during the distraction phase of the osteotomy [1, 8]. Proximal to the tibial tubercule, patellar tendon should be identified and protected from the possible damage that might be caused by the blade of the saw by placing a broad retractor anteriorly. It is of high importance to conduct careful subperiosteal dissections in order to protect and secure the posterior neurovascular structures.

After the subperiosteal dissection and exposure of the entire proximal-medial portion of the tibia, a guide wire is inserted, starting proximal to the tibial tubercule and aiming toward the tip of the fibular head with an anteromedial to posterolateral trajectory. After the insertion of the first guide wire, it is optional to place another wire posteriorly to determine the osteotomy's sagittal angle that can influence the amount of the sagittal slope. If a reduction of the posterior tibial slope is desired, the posterior guide wire should be placed more superiorly resulting in a flatter cut. If a rise of the sagittal slope is desired, then the posterior guidewire should be placed more inferiorly.

An oscillating saw is used to make the first cut of the osteotomy on the anteromedial cortex.

This cut is advanced with osteotomes until to a distance of 1–1.5 cm to the lateral cortex of the tibia, in order not to cause any fracture on the tibial plateau. In addition to that, it is also recommended, that the vertical distance from the tip of the osteotome to the lateral tibial plateau should be 1.25 times of the horizontal distance to the lateral tibial cortex, to minimize the risk of any fracture on the lateral tibial plateau. Hereby, the osteotomy is ended, followed by the opening of the osteotomized bone and very gentle and careful application of valgus force on the tibia. Osteotomy side is opened sequentially with calibrated wedges. As a result of that, a new mechanical axis has been reconstructed (**Figure 4**). The new mechanical axis is confirmed by either placing a cord of electrocautery or a long alignment rod from the center of the hip to the center of the ankle and confirming its distance from the knee joint under image intensifier. It was also suggested to add a concomitant tibial tuberosity osteotomy, if more than 12.5 mm correction is required, in order to avoid the potentially adverse effects of patella baja and increased pressure in patellofemoral compartment [8, 39].

The advantages of the medial open wedge osteotomy can be summarized as:

- the ability to provide biplanar correction and biplanar alignment (coronal and sagittal),
- no limb shortening,
- no bone loss,
- no need for fibular osteotomy,

- use of a single cut with no need to detach the muscles,
- little risk of peroneal nerve injury,
- ability to adjust the amount of correction during surgery,
- easier conversion to arthroplasty.

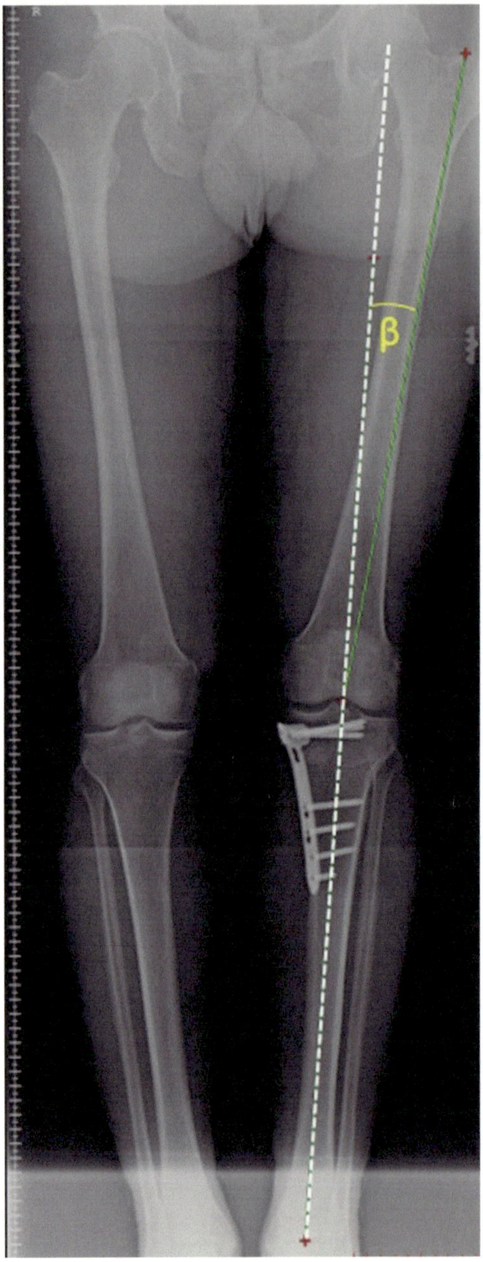

Figure 4.
Post-operative weight-bearing orthoroentgenogram of a patient after MOWHTO. β (7° in this case) is the angle formed by the anatomical axis of femur and the weight-bearing axis (white dashed line) or the mechanical and anatomical axes of tibia, where all three axes are overlapping each other in the tibia.

The disadvantages of the medial open wedge osteotomy can be summarized as:

- the need for bone graft,
- the risk of delayed union or non-union.

8.1.1 Fixation of the medial open wedge osteotomy

Plate fixation was reported to be biomechanically superior as compared to external fixation [40, 41]. Plates without spacer wedges were shown to have higher rates of failure compared to those with wedges [11, 41]. Plate fixators (i.e., The TomoFix plate) are manufactured with the principles of the locking compression plate (LCP) concept; meanwhile offering the advantage of a rigid fixation, and providing early weight-bearing, and early start of motion while the normal pre-operative posterior tibial slope is maintained [13, 14, 42]. TomoFix plates (Synthes, West Chester, PA) and Puddu plates (Arthrex, Naples, FL) were detected to provide adequate biomechanical stability, whereas in case of lateral cortex fracture, TomoFix plates were detected to provide adequate stability without the need of any additional lateral fixation [8, 42]. The biomechanics of three spacer plates with different length was studied, while two were with locking bolts, and one was the TomoFix plate, which was shown to be superior at single load-to-failure and cyclical load-to-failure tests and also possessed the maximum residual stability after failure of the lateral cortex, in addition to least motion at the osteotomy gap [43–45].

8.1.2 Bone healing after the medial open wedge osteotomy

After medial open wedge HTO procedure, healing was shown to start from the lateral hinge and advancing toward the medial aspect, while 3 months after the procedure, callus formation, and ossification was visible [8, 11, 13]. In our clinical practice, 6 months post-operatively more than 80% of the gap is filled with newly formed bone (**Figure 5**), and more than 80% of patients X-ray and CT scan, a consolidation is visible at the end of the first post-operative year.

8.1.3 Spacers and autografts for the medial open wedge osteotomy

To enhance stability and accelerate the healing, we like many other surgeons prefer to fill the gap of osteotomy with grafts or bone substitutes. Post-operative alignment and clinical outcome were reported to be comparable between beta-tricalcium phosphate (TCP) and hydroxyapatite (HAp), but TCP was noted to possess a significant superiority regarding osteoconductivity and bioabsorbability after 18 months [46]. After the TomoFix plate removal, it was observed, that TCP was completely absorbed and the newly forming bone was completely remodeled and incorporated into osteotomized tibia [47].

Autogenous iliac bone graft as the bone filler is widely used at the end of the HTO procedure. It is also considered as a reliable bone filler in patients who are at risk of non-/delayed union such as smokers, obese patients, and those with [48]. Results with autograft were reported to be superior with lower rates of total complications as compared to allograft and bone substitutes such as the calcium-phosphate ceramic spacer [49].

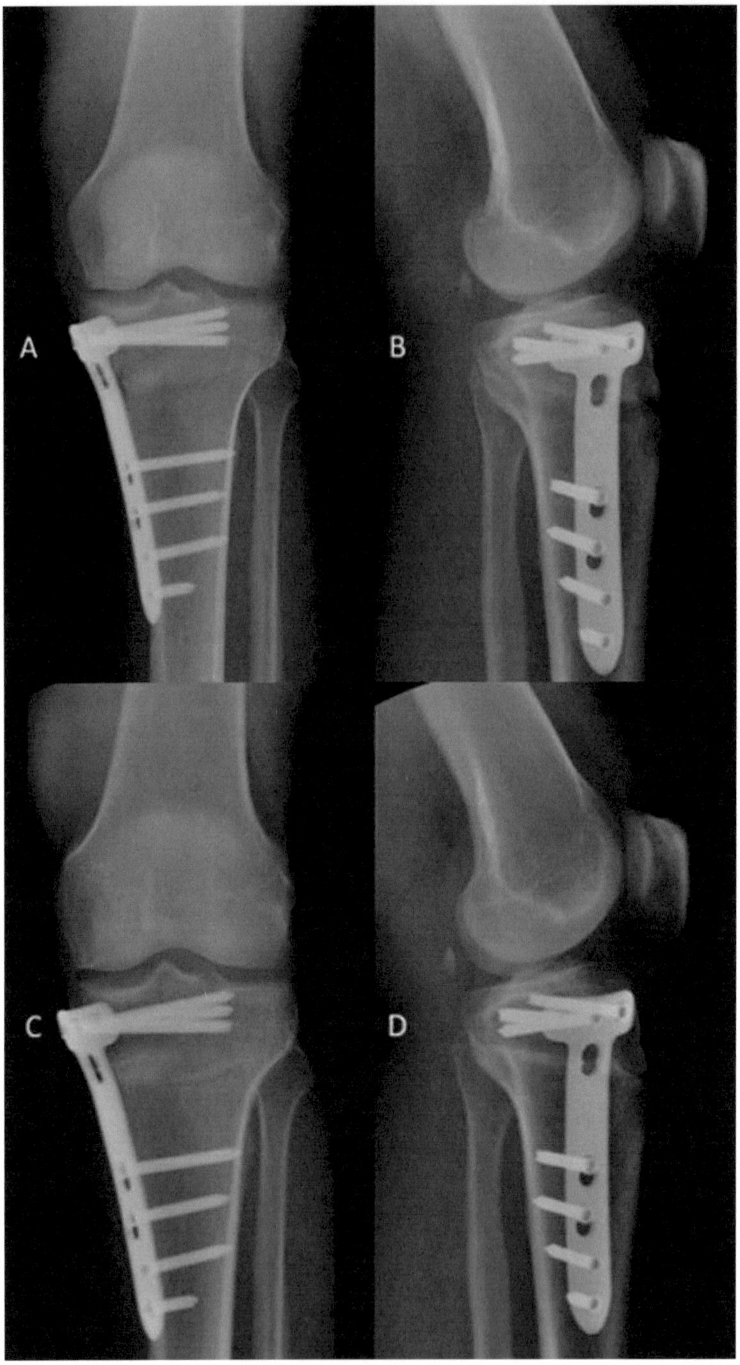

Figure 5.
Anteroposterior and lateral X-rays of the patient after 6 weeks (A and B) and 6 months (C and D) post-operatively.

8.2 Lateral closing wedge osteotomy

Lateral closing wedge osteotomy (LCWO) starts with an inverted L-shaped incision directed anterolaterally, while the vertical part is placed on the lateral edge of the tibial tubercule and the horizontal part is placed 1–1.5 cm distally to lateral knee joint line. This osteotomy requires peroneal nerve exposure and dissection, which is found on the anatomical area located the 2–3 cm distally to fibular proximal styloid process and crossing the neck of the fibula. The nerve should be carefully dissected and protected. After the dissection and protection of the peroneal nerve, the anterior compartment muscles are elevated subperiosteally from the anterolateral aspect of tibia while the incision is advanced distally. Patellar tendon should be protected while placing a retractor between the tendon and the anterior tibia. Following this

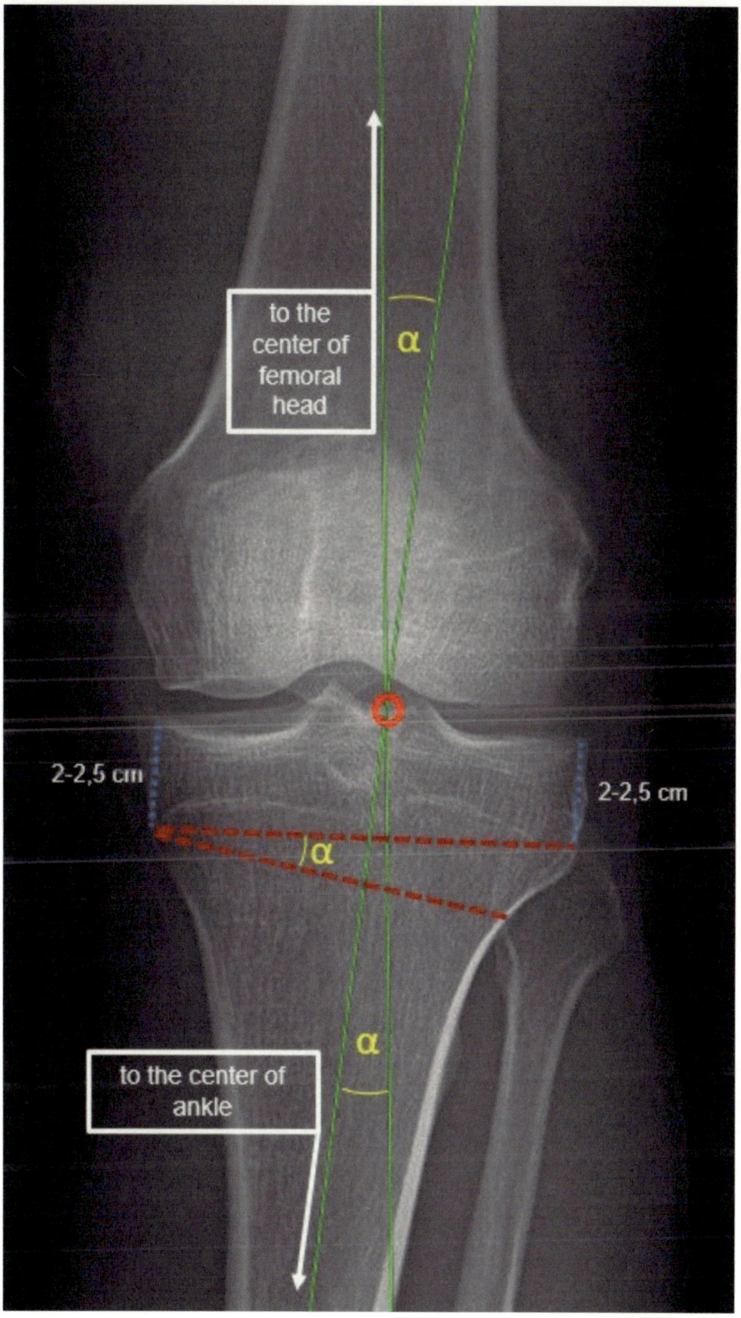

Figure 6.
Pre-operative planning for LCWHTO. α, the correction angle, is the angle formed by the mechanical axes of femur and tibia that are aimed to be provided post-operatively. The osteotomy lines are drawn as red dashed lines.

step, the tibiofibular joint can be disrupted by using an osteotome, combined with the resection of the medial one-third of fibula or applying a fibular shaft osteotomy placed 10 cm distally to the fibular head. After that, we usually identify the joint by using two needles and placing the osteotomy guide parallel to the needles aiming 2–2.5 cm distal to the joint line. Following this step, the osteotomy guide is secured to the bone by using two smooth pins, over which the plate is also placed with high precision to the bone while directing it exactly parallel to the posterior slope of the tibial. Before starting to perform with the osteotomy by using an oscillating saw and osteotomes, posterior neurovascular structures, and patellar tendon should be ensured to be protected by the retractors. It is important to end the tip of the osteotome with a distance of 1 cm from the medial tibial cortex and 2–2.5 cm distal to the knee joint line (**Figure 6**). With the help of the osteotomy guide, the required amount of bone can be resected. This step is followed by the application of the plate over the previously placed pins that are replaced with screws. By using a large reduction clamp, the osteotomy is closed and compressed, followed by the insertion of the remaining screws.

8.3 Dome osteotomy

A dome osteotomy is usually indicated when a correction more than 20° are needed. The osteotomy is performed by applying an inverted U-shaped (dome shaped) osteotomy proximal to tibial tubercule. Especially in cases with accompanying patellofemoral disease, by staying proximal to tibial tubercule, distal tibia is shifted anteriorly, yielding to anterior translation of the tibial tubercule, which maintains the patellar height. After the placement of a jig, anteroposterior drill holes are applied in a half barrel shaped configuration while staying proximal to tibial tubercule. During dome osteotomy a partial resection of the fibular shaft might be necessary. Before starting with the osteotomy, the amount of correction should be certainly indicated on the jig and marked with Steinmann pins located in the proximal and distal fragments. Removal of the jig is followed by careful osteotomizing of the posterior cortex, while the pre-determined amount of correction is achieved by anteriorization of the distal fragment together with the tibial tubercule. Dome osteotomy is usually fixed by using an external fixator. Increased operative time, patient discomfort caused by the external fixator, possible risks of pin tract infections, need for frequent follow-up visits for the fine-tuning of external fixator or assessment of the wound side are the disadvantages of dome osteotomy. In our clinical practice, we do not apply the dome osteotomy frequently as a result of the aforementioned disadvantages, while we spare this procedure for patients requiring high degrees of bony correction.

9. Survival rates of high tibial osteotomy

A good surgical technique combined with rigid fixation together with meticulous patient selection and appropriate post-operative rehabilitation protocols are keys to long-term survival of HTO. Koshino et al. reported 93.2% as the 10-year survival rate for closed wedge osteotomy, related to some post operation factors including, valgus anatomical angle of 10°, no flexion contracture and concomitant patellofemoral decompression procedure if indicated [50]. In patients who underwent medial open wedge high tibial osteotomy a 10-year delay of arthroplasty in 63% of 73 patients [51], and in 85% of 203 patients was shown [52].

In a study of 54 patients with osteoarthritis limited to medial compartment, 24% rate of conversion to arthroplasty was reported after a median of 16.5 years with either medial opening or lateral closing wedge HTO, while no significant difference regarding the functional scores and survival rates was found between the two techniques [53].

It was reported, that authors showed that the lateral closing wedge osteotomy was related to higher number of conversion to total joint replacement, whereas the medial opening wedge HTO was related to higher incidence of complications [54].

Results of HTO were noted to be good within the first 10 years following the surgery; whereas, a worsening of the results was also shown after 15 years [55, 56].

10. Complications

HTO's complication rate was reported between 7 and 55%. It should be remembered that HTO requires a long learning curve leading to decreased rates of complication [1, 7, 8].

With more experience and over the course of years, rates of complications were decreased to 8–15% [1].

It is a fact that medial opening wedge HTO became more popular that the other techniques, because of the successful outcomes. Complications including hardware failure, hardware irritation (up to 40%), loss of correction, non-union, lateral tibial plateau fractures, medial collateral ligament injuries were reported for opening wedge HTO [1, 8, 57]. In addition to that, lateral cortex violation was reports as an important factor for fixation failure, resulting in a minimum 4° of loss of correction in the final follow-up as compared to immediate post-operative X-rays [49]. In a study comprising 100 consecutive MOWHTO patients with an average follow-up of 4 years, allograft combined with plasma-rich platelets and/or DBM was associated with the risk of non-union [58]. Severe adverse events were reported to be seen more common as a result of HTO in patients with diabetes, active smoking, displaced lateral hinge fractures, and patients with no compliance [59].

11. High tibial osteotomy combined with concurrent cartilage procedures

HTO with and without articular cartilage procedures or meniscus allograft transplantation was evaluated in a systematic review assessed and concluded that HTO combined with cartilage procedures led to excellent short-term and mid-term survival and good clinical outcomes, while deterioration was detected after 10 years [60]. Another study of 43 patients with HTO and ACI showed long-term, improved cartilage survival, and a decreased rate of revision in patients with mild varus deformity (<5°) of knee joint [61]. HTO was intended to preserve the joint and chondral surfaces as much as possible to delay the time interval until total knee arthroplasty. In order to be successful and preserve the joint as much as possible, we also prefer to apply concurrent cartilage procedure to delay the TKA as much as possible.

12. Results of high tibial osteotomy

La Prade et al. reported about the modified Cincinnati Knee Scores (CKS) in patients younger than 55 years old who underwent HTO for medial OA and varus deformity in a single surgeon study from 2000 to 2007. They had strict inclusion and exclusion criteria which excluded patients undergoing additional procedures or treatments. Each patient was applied an offloading brace pre-operatively. If the patient did not get symptom relief, they were not offered a HTO. Forty-seven patients were available for follow-up. The CKS improved from 42.9 to 65.1 ($P < 0.0001$). Function subscore improved from 24.2 to 34.2 ($P < 0.001$). Functional score improved significantly at 6 weeks, 1 and 2 years [62].

Howells et al. reviewed 164 consecutive patients that underwent lateral closing wedge HTO between 2000 and 2002. Among them, 100 patients met the inclusion criteria and had a follow-up duration of 5–10 years post-operatively. Data were collected prospectively; however, the study reviewed the data retrospectively. To assess outcome WOMAC and KSS were used. At 5 years, 87% of survival rate was reported with the remainder undergoing TKA. This rate dropped to 79% after 10 at 10 years. It was detected that those requiring revision to TKA had a significantly lower WOMAC score (47 vs. 65, $P < 0.001$), were older (54 years old vs. 49, $P = 0.006$) and had a higher BMI (30.2 vs. 27.9, $P = 0.005$). They concluded that a patient less than 55 years old, with a BMI less than 30 and a pre-operative WOMAC score of >45, were positive predictors regarding failure. The authors underlined the importance of using of pre- operative functional scores to use in the decision-making process [63].

Conflict of interest

The authors declare no conflict of interest.

Author details

Tuna Pehlivanoglu[1,2], Kerem Yildirim[3,4] and Tahsin Beyzadeoglu[3,5]*

1 Department of Orthopedic Surgery and Traumatology, EMSEY Hospital, Istanbul, Turkey

2 Faculty of Health Sciences, Yeni Yuzyil University, Istanbul, Turkey

3 Beyzadeoglu Clinic, Istanbul, Turkey

4 Faculty of Health Sciences, Istanbul Gelisim University, Istanbul, Turkey

5 Faculty of Health Sciences, Halic University, Istanbul, Turkey

*Address all correspondence to: tbeyzade@superonline.com

References

[1] Amendola A, Bonasia DE. Results of high tibial osteotomy: Review of the literature. International Orthopaedics. 2010;**34**:155-160

[2] Jackson JP, Waugh W. Tibial osteotomy for osteoarthritis of the knee. Journal of Bone and Joint Surgery. British Volume (London). 1961;**43-B**:746-751

[3] Jackson JP, Waugh W. The technique and complications of upper tibial osteotomy. A review of 226 operations. Journal of Bone and Joint Surgery. British Volume (London). 1974;**56**:236-245

[4] Coventry MB. Proximal tibial varus osteotomy for osteoarthritis of the lateral compartment of the knee. The Journal of Bone and Joint Surgery. American Volume. 1987;**69**:32-38

[5] Hernigou P, Medevielle D, Debeyre J, et al. Proximal tibial osteotomy for osteoarthritis with varus deformity. A ten to thirteen-year follow-up study. The Journal of Bone and Joint Surgery. American Volume. 1987;**69**:332-354

[6] Debeyre J, Patte D. Value of corrective osteotomies in the treatment of certain knee diseases with axial deviation. Revue du Rhumatisme et des Maladies Ostéo-Articulaires. 1962;**29**:722-729

[7] Aglietti P, Buzzi R, Vena LM, et al. High tibial valgus osteotomy for medial gonarthrosis: A 10- to 21-year study. The Journal of Knee Surgery. 2003;**16**:21-26

[8] Lee DC, Byun SJ. High tibial osteotomy. Knee Surgery & Related Research. 2012;**24**:61-69

[9] Lash NJ, Feller JA, Batty LM, et al. Bone grafts and bone substitutes for opening-wedge osteotomies of the knee: A systematic review. Arthroscopy. 2015;**31**:720-730

[10] Saragaglia D, Blaysat M, Inman D, et al. Outcome of opening wedge high tibial osteotomy augmented with a biosorb(R) wedge and fixed with a plate and screws in 124 patients with a mean of ten years follow-up. International Orthopaedics. 2011;**35**:1151-1156

[11] Sabzevari S, Ebrahimpour A, Roudi MK, et al. High tibial osteotomy: A systematic review and current concept. Archives of Bone and Joint Surgery. 2016;**4**:204-212

[12] Lobenhoffer P, Agneskirchner JD. Improvements in surgical technique of valgus high tibial osteotomy. Knee Surgery, Sports Traumatology, Arthroscopy. 2003;**11**:132-138

[13] Staubli AE, De Simoni C, Babst R, et al. TomoFix: A new LCP concept for open wedge osteotomy of the medial proximal tibia—Early results in 92 cases. Injury. 2003;**34**(Suppl 2):B55-B62

[14] Niemeyer P, Schmal H, Hauschild O, et al. Open-wedge osteotomy using an internal plate fixator in patients with medial-compartment gonarthritis and varus malalignment: 3-year results with regard to preoperative arthroscopic and radiographic findings. Arthroscopy. 2010;**26**:1607-1616

[15] Sommer C, Gautier E, Muller M, et al. First clinical results of the locking compression plate (LCP). Injury. 2003;**34**(Suppl 2):B43-B54

[16] Akamatsu Y, Koshino T, Saito T, et al. Changes in osteosclerosis of the osteoarthritic knee after high tibial osteotomy. Clinical Orthopaedics and Related Research. 1997;**334**:207-214

[17] Takahashi S, Tomihisa K, Saito T. Decrease of osteosclerosis

in subchondral bone of medial compartmental osteoarthritic knee seven to nineteen years after high tibial valgus osteotomy. Bulletin/Hospital for Joint Diseases. 2002-2003;**61**(1-2):58-62

[18] Jung W-H, Takeuchi R, Chun C-W, et al. Second-look arthroscopic assessment of cartilage regeneration after medial opening-wedge high tibial osteotomy. Arthroscopy. 2014;**30**:72-79

[19] Holden DL, James SL, Larson RL, et al. Proximal tibial osteotomy in patients who are fifty years old or less. A long-term follow-up study. The Journal of Bone and Joint Surgery. American Volume. 1988;**70**:977-982

[20] Odenbring S, Tjornstrand B, Egund N, et al. Function after tibial osteotomy for medial gonarthrosis below aged 50 years. Acta Orthopaedica Scandinavica. 1989;**60**:527-531

[21] Khoshbin A, Sheth U, Ogilvie-Harris D, et al. The effect of patient, provider and surgical factors on survivorship of high tibial osteotomy to total knee arthroplasty: A population-based study. Knee Surgery, Sports Traumatology, Arthroscopy. 2017;**25**:887-894

[22] Preston CF, Fulkerson EW, Meislin R, et al. Osteotomy about the knee: Applications, techniques, and results. The Journal of Knee Surgery. 2005;**18**:258-272

[23] Brinkman J-M, Lobenhoffer P, Agneskirchner JD, et al. Osteotomies around the knee: Patient selection, stability of fixation and bone healing in high tibial osteotomies. Journal of Bone and Joint Surgery. British Volume (London). 2008;**90**:1548-1557

[24] Rossi R, Bonasia DE, Amendola A. The role of high tibial osteotomy in the varus knee. The Journal of the American Academy of Orthopaedic Surgeons. 2011;**19**:590-599

[25] Phillips CL, Silver DAT, Schranz PJ, et al. The measurement of patellar height: A review of the methods of imaging. Journal of Bone and Joint Surgery. British Volume (London). 2010;**92**:1045-1053

[26] Babis GC, An K-N, Chao EYS, et al. Double level osteotomy of the knee: A method to retain joint-line obliquity. Clinical results. The Journal of Bone and Joint Surgery. American Volume. 2002;**84**:1380-1388

[27] Coventry MB, Ilstrup DM, Wallrichs SL. Proximal tibial osteotomy. A critical long-term study of eighty-seven cases. The Journal of Bone and Joint Surgery. American Volume. 1993;**75**:196-201

[28] Bonasia DE, Dettoni F, Sito G, et al. Medial opening wedge high tibial osteotomy for medial compartment overload/arthritis in the varus knee: Prognostic factors. The American Journal of Sports Medicine. 2014;**42**:690-698

[29] Hsu RW, Himeno S, Coventry MB, et al. Normal axial alignment of the lower extremity and load-bearing distribution at the knee. Clinical Orthopaedics and Related Research. 1990;**255**:215-227

[30] Moreland JR, Bassett LW, Hanker GJ. Radiographic analysis of the axial alignment of the lower extremity. The Journal of Bone and Joint Surgery. American Volume. 1987;**69**:745-749

[31] Tetsworth K, Paley D. Malalignment and degenerative arthropathy. The Orthopedic Clinics of North America. 1994;**25**:367-377

[32] Fujisawa Y, Masuhara K, Shiomi S. The effect of high tibial osteotomy on osteoarthritis of the knee. An arthroscopic study of 54 knee joints. The Orthopedic Clinics of North America. 1979;**10**:585-608

[33] Iorio R, Healy WL. Unicompartmental arthritis of the knee. The Journal of Bone and Joint Surgery. American Volume. 2003;**85**:1351-1364

[34] Coventry MB. Upper tibial osteotomy for gonarthrosis. The evolution of the operation in the last 18 years and long term results. The Orthopedic Clinics of North America. 1979;**10**:191-210

[35] Coventry MB, Bowman PW. Long-term results of upper tibial osteotomy for degenerative arthritis of the knee. Acta Orthopaedica Belgica. 1982;**48**:139-156

[36] Smith TO, Sexton D, Mitchell P, et al. Opening- or closing-wedged high tibial osteotomy: A meta-analysis of clinical and radiological outcomes. The Knee. 2011;**18**:361-368

[37] Dugdale TW, Noyes FR, Styer D. Preoperative planning for high tibial osteotomy. The effect of lateral tibiofemoral separation and tibiofemoral length. Clinical Orthopaedics and Related Research. 1992;**274**:248-264

[38] Muller M, Strecker W. Arthroscopy prior to osteotomy around the knee? Archives of Orthopaedic and Trauma Surgery. 2008;**128**:1217-1221

[39] McNamara I, Birmingham TB, Fowler PJ, et al. High tibial osteotomy: Evolution of research and clinical applications—A Canadian experience. Knee Surgery, Sports Traumatology, Arthroscopy. 2013;**21**:23-31

[40] Zhim F, Laflamme GY, Viens H, et al. Biomechanical stability of high tibial opening wedge osteotomy: Internal fixation versus external fixation. Clinical Biomechanics (Bristol, Avon). 2005;**20**:871-876

[41] Spahn G, Muckley T, Kahl E, et al. Biomechanical investigation of different internal fixations in medial opening-wedge high tibial osteotomy. Clinical Biomechanics (Bristol, Avon). 2006;**21**:272-278

[42] Stoffel K, Stachowiak G, Kuster M. Open wedge high tibial osteotomy: biomechanical investigation of the modified Arthrex Osteotomy Plate (Puddu Plate) and the TomoFix Plate. Clinical Biomechanics (Bristol, Avon). 2004;**19**:944-950

[43] Pape D, Kohn D, van Giffen N, et al. Differences in fixation stability between spacer plate and plate fixator following high tibial osteotomy. Knee Surgery, Sports Traumatology, Arthroscopy. 2013;**21**:82-89

[44] Kyung H-S, Lee B-J, Kim J-W, et al. Biplanar open wedge high tibial osteotomy in the medial compartment osteoarthritis of the knee joint: Comparison between the Aescula and TomoFix plate. Clinics in Orthopedic Surgery. 2015;7:185-190

[45] Golovakhsmall A, Maxim LC, Orljanski W, Benedetto K-P, et al. Comparison of theoretical fixation stability of three devices employed in medial opening wedge high tibial osteotomy: A finite element analysis. BMC Musculoskeletal Disorders. 2014;**15**:230

[46] Onodera J, Kondo E, Omizu N, et al. Beta-tricalcium phosphate shows superior absorption rate and osteoconductivity compared to hydroxyapatite in open-wedge high tibial osteotomy. Knee Surgery, Sports Traumatology, Arthroscopy. 2014;**22**:2763-2770

[47] Gaasbeek RDA, Toonen HG, van Heerwaarden RJ, et al. Mechanism of bone incorporation of beta-TCP bone substitute in open wedge tibial osteotomy in patients. Biomaterials. 2005;**26**:6713-6719

[48] Meidinger G, Imhoff AB, Paul J, et al. May smokers and overweight patients be treated with a medial open-wedge HTO? Risk factors for non-union. Knee Surgery, Sports Traumatology, Arthroscopy. 2011;**19**:333-339

[49] Kuremsky MA, Schaller TM, Hall CC, et al. Comparison of autograft vs allograft in opening-wedge high tibial osteotomy. The Journal of Arthroplasty. 2010;**25**:951-957

[50] Koshino T, Yoshida T, Ara Y, et al. Fifteen to twenty-eight years' follow-up results of high tibial valgus osteotomy for osteoarthritic knee. The Knee. 2004;**11**:439-444

[51] Weale AE, Lee AS, MacEachern AG. High tibial osteotomy using a dynamic axial external fixator. Clinical Orthopaedics and Related Research. 2001;**382**:154-167

[52] Hernigou P, Ma W. Open wedge tibial osteotomy with acrylic bone cement as bone substitute. The Knee. 2001;**8**:103-110

[53] Schallberger A, Jacobi M, Wahl P, et al. High tibial valgus osteotomy in unicompartmental medial osteoarthritis of the knee: A retrospective follow-up study over 13-21 years. Knee Surgery, Sports Traumatology, Arthroscopy. 2011;**19**:122-127

[54] Duivenvoorden T, Brouwer RW, Baan A, et al. Comparison of closing-wedge and opening-wedge high tibial osteotomy for medial compartment osteoarthritis of the knee: A randomized controlled trial with a six-year follow-up. The Journal of Bone and Joint Surgery. American Volume. 2014;**96**:1425-1432

[55] Akizuki S, Shibakawa A, Takizawa T, et al. The long-term outcome of high tibial osteotomy: A ten- to 20-year follow-up. Journal of Bone and Joint Surgery. British Volume (London). 2008;**90**:592-596

[56] Billings A, Scott DF, Camargo MP, et al. High tibial osteotomy with a calibrated osteotomy guide, rigid internal fixation, and early motion. Long-term follow-up. The Journal of Bone and Joint Surgery. American Volume. 2000;**82**:70-79

[57] Dewilde TR, Dauw J, Vandenneucker H, et al. Opening wedge distal femoral varus osteotomy using the Puddu plate and calcium phosphate bone cement. Knee Surgery, Sports Traumatology, Arthroscopy. 2013;**21**:249-254

[58] Giuseffi SA, Replogle WH, Shelton WR. Opening-wedge high tibial osteotomy: Review of 100 consecutive cases. Arthroscopy. 2015;**31**:2128-2137

[59] Martin R, Birmingham TB, Willits K, et al. Adverse event rates and classifications in medial opening wedge high tibial osteotomy. The American Journal of Sports Medicine. 2014;**42**:1118-1126

[60] Harris JD, McNeilan R, Siston RA, et al. Survival and clinical outcome of isolated high tibial osteotomy and combined biological knee reconstruction. The Knee. 2013;**20**:154-161

[61] Bode G, Schmal H, Pestka JM, et al. A non-randomized controlled clinical trial on autologous chondrocyte implantation (ACI) in cartilage defects of the medial femoral condyle with or without high tibial osteotomy in patients with varus deformity of less than 5 degrees. Archives of Orthopaedic and Trauma Surgery. 2013;**133**:43-49

[62] Laprade RF, Spiridonov SI, Nystrom LM, et al. Prospective outcomes of young and middle-aged adults with medial compartment osteoarthritis

treated with a proximal tibial opening wedge osteotomy. Arthroscopy. 2012;**28**:354-364

[63] Howells NR, Salmon L, Waller A, et al. The outcome at ten years of lateral closing-wedge high tibial osteotomy: Determinants of survival and functional outcome. The Bone & Joint Journal. 2014;**96-B**:1491-1497